SMEAR

SMEAR TESTS

Every woman's guide

Dr Jane Chomet
and Julian Chomet

Thorsons
An Imprint of HarperCollinsPublishers

Thorsons
An Imprint of HarperCollins*Publishers*
77-85 Fulham Palace Road,
Hammersmith, London W6 8JB

First published by Thorsons as *Cervical Cancer* 1989
This revised new format edition 1991
· 3 5 7 9 10 8 6 4 2

© 1989 Dr Jane Chomet and Julian Chomet
Illustrations by Peter Gardiner, photographs by Sara Furse and
Frank Netter, Ciba Geigy

Dr Jane Chomet and Julian Chomet assert the moral right to
be identified as the authors of this work

A catalogue record for this book
is available from the British Library

ISBN 0 7225 2500 1

Typesetting by MJL Limited, Hitchin, Hertfordshire
Printed in Great Britain by
HarperCollinsManufacturing Glasgow

About the authors

DR JANE CHOMET is a medical practitioner. Her interest in cervical cancer was kindled in the early sixties by Dr George Papanicolaou, the inventor of the cervical smear test, who visited the Royal Free Hospital when she was a student there.

Since then she has screened women in her practice, taught other doctors to take smears, and introduced the first general practice-based colposcopy service in Britain.

Julian Chomet, M.Sc. in biological sciences, has worked as a medical journalist for *General Practitioner* newspaper. Since 1984 he has worked as a freelance journalist, author and documentary writer/director, specializing in scientific and medical topics.

Mother and son joined forces to write this book together.

Acknowledgements

WE WOULD LIKE TO THANK Mr Patrick Walker, consultant gynaecologist at the Royal Free Hospital, London, for his invaluable help and advice in the preparation of this book. We also wish to thank Mr Daniel Falkner for providing the coffee and cakes, photocopying and ferrying around various versions of the manuscript, and displaying remarkable good humour in the face of the authors' invading his weekends for the best part of a year. Also deserving of thanks is Jane Stephens, librarian at the Whittington Hospital, London.

Contents

Foreword

WE HAVE ALL KNOWN or know of someone who will die of cancer. In most cases it is a long drawn out and painful experience for everybody concerned. There is little hope of a cure and survival is often only a matter of months or years, with the permanent and very real fear of a reoccurrence. The big 'C' still fills us with a primitive fear. Fear not just of dying, but of the terrible way cancer kills its victims and the way it makes the victims feel afraid and outcast. People are *still* embarrassed to say: 'I have cancer.'

Fear and embarrassment is what this wonderful book is trying to eradicate with a message of *hope*. It is a positive book with a positive message: don't be embarrassed, don't be lazy; *do* something to prevent it, because you can.

Most forms of cancer cannot be detected early and certainly cannot be tested for on a regular basis with any ease. Here we have information for men and women about cervical cancer, which we can prevent, or if detected early, we can cure (a word still not often associated with cancer).

It is our responsibility to protect our partners and inform our children. There is no need to be ignorant, to carry with us still this Victorian attitude towards our 'private parts'. There is a generation of women who would never dream of going for a smear test because it would embarrass them.

Here is an important, honest book, that manages to be both

9

interesting and informative, a help to generations of women, who I hope will not in future die of embarrassment — or ignorance. It has been written by an extraordinary woman, a true pioneer in her field, together with her son Julian, who is a scientific and medical journalist. It's an important and positive piece of knowledge — it's here, it's available and we can have a choice in this one area of our lives. Let's choose life.

Felicity Kendal
London
1988

Introduction

THE WORD CANCER is an emotive one. For many years cancer was synonymous with death; the detection of the disease was usually at a late stage and the treatments were few and, for the most part, able only to relieve the suffering a little.

During the last two decades, however, there have been enormous advances in the methods of detection as well as in the treatment of cancer. With the most modern screening techniques it is now possible to detect and to treat potential cancer of the cervix in its pre-cancerous state. Cervical cancer is therefore perfectly curable in its early stages, which is why it is so very important that both women and men — who also have an important role to play — be informed about it.

The disease itself is symptomless and by the time it manifests itself has usually progressed to an advanced stage. It begins as a pre-cancerous change in the cells of the cervix and, if undetected, will spread from the cervix to the nearby organs and then throughout the woman's body.

The test used to identify the disease — the cervical (or Pap) smear — is simple, quick and painless. Pre-cancerous or cancerous changes can be detected by examining a few cells taken from the skin of the cervix. If diseased tissue is discovered, it is usually easily removed and a lifetime of freedom from cancer is then a reasonable expectation.

Any and every woman, including virginal women, may be

affected by cervical cancer and it may develop at any time of her life. It is a cancer whose prevalence has been steadily increasing, but only in recent years has there been any significant research and development in the treatment of the disease. In addition, social taboos and prejudices have encouraged both sexes to regard cervical cancer as a 'dirty' disease, one linked solely to promiscuity. Research has now shown that this is, in fact, not the case and it is to be hoped that more women will now present themselves for screening and that funds will now be available throughout the world for more regular cervical smears.

Recent research has indicated that certain bacteria and viruses which may exist in the semen of some men could cause cancerous changes in the cervix, making it possible for sexual partners to unwittingly transmit potentially carcinogenic infections to each other. The latest research into the viruses which have been implicated in causing cervical cancer is examined in the book, as are all the measures that both men and women can take to protect themselves.

Since cervical cancer is symptomless until the later and more dangerous stages it cannot be emphasized enough that women should be checked when they seem to be well. If every woman had a cervical smear once a year and each examination were perfectly performed, the results were correctly reported and each woman reached in time and the treatment promptly carried out, no woman would ever die of cervical cancer.

The key to fighting the disease lies mainly with women themselves, but also to a great extent with men, and this is something we will discuss in some detail later in the book. We have tried to explain the nature of cervical cancer, how it affects women, who is likely to transmit and be attacked by the disease and how it can be detected and subsequently treated. Our hope is that the information contained in the book will help save lives, not only among readers but perhaps also the friends and relatives of readers.

Chapter 1

The history of cervical cancer

- Cervical cancer is not a new disease. It has been around for thousands of years.

- The link between sexual intercourse and cervical cancer was suggested more than one hundred years ago.

- Cervical cancer is the second most common cancer of women after breast cancer.

- Of an estimated 460,000 new cases of cervical cancer each year, around 75 per cent are in the developing world.

- Between 60 and 90 per cent of women dying from invasive cancer have never had a smear, and in some areas in the developing world this figure is even higher.

- The early form of cervical cancer, cervical pre-cancer, is on the increase throughout the world.

Human beings have always had to face the risks associated with sexual intercourse and one of these is cervical cancer. Around 4500 BC it was recognized by the third Egyptian dynasty. The great Greek doctor and philosopher, Hippocrates, was one of the first to mention cervical cancer specifically some six thousand years ago. Later, around 100 AD, Soranus of Ephesus, one of the leading authorities on gynaecology in the ancient world, gave a detailed description of the female genital organs, identifying the cervix and its cancerous conditions. Between 500 and 575

AD, Aetius of Armida, physician to the Roman Emperor Justinian I, and a prolific author on midwifery and women's diseases, described the cancer with these words, 'The tumour was usually at the cervix, hard, resistant and uneven to touch. From it came a thin watery discharge reddish in colour'.

Powerful and convincing evidence that cervical cancer was sexually transmitted, came in the 19th century from the statistics of Professor Domenico Rigoni-Stern, chief physician of a hospital in Verona. In 1842, he described the frequency and occurrence of cervical cancer among married and widowed women, and the rarity of the disease in virginal women. Since then, various epidemiological studies on cultural, ethnic and social groups of populations have highlighted certain behavioural, social, and occupational aspects of men and women which have significant bearing upon the epidemiology of this disease.

A worldwide disease

Cervical cancer is the second most common cancer among women in the world, second only to breast cancer. In Africa, central and tropical South America, China, India and other Asian countries, it is the most common cancer among women. In North America and Europe it is the fourth most common cancer. Globally (see Table 1) there are around 460,000 new cases of cervical cancer (not pre-cancer) each year. Around 77 per cent of these occur in the developing countries, a reflection of poor screening and treatment facilities. Approximately 16 per cent of the world total occurs in India.

Figures from the developed countries suggest that mortality from cervical cancer has declined by approximately 30 per cent between 1960 and 1980, with early diagnosis through screening and prompt treatment being a major factor in its decline. In some nations the mortality rate has been reduced by up to 60 per cent. However, it is difficult to get precise figures from developing countries because cancer data in general is often incomplete.

The overall incidence of the invasive disease (i.e which has gone beyond the skin of the cervix) has fallen slightly but a disturbingly high proportion of cases now occurs in women under 35 years of age with an increase of 6 per cent within the last ten years. There have also been reports showing an increase in the speed of progression and aggression of the disease from the precancerous to the cancerous stage. Between 60 and 90 per cent of women who die of invasive cervical cancer have *never* had a smear.

Table 1 Estimated annual number of new cases of cervical cancer

Regions	No. of new cases
North America	15,700
Latin America	44,000
Europe	47,200
USSR	31,300
Africa	36,900
China	131,500
India	71,600
Japan	9,700
Asia (other parts)	70,300
Australia/New Zealand	1,200
Developed regions	105,100
Developing regions	354,300
Total	459,400

Source: Bulletin of the World Health Organization 64 (4) 607-618 (1986).

Chapter 2

Cervical cancer — where, what, why?

- The cervix is a part (neck) of the womb found deep in the vagina and is affected by changes in hormonal levels.

- The cervix plays an important role in sexual function and reproduction by facilitating sperm transport to the ovum (egg), lubricating the vagina for intercourse, and holding the pregnancy in the uterus.

- The transformation zone, where the two types of cervical skin meet, is the prime site in which pre-cancerous changes occur most frequently.

- Human papilloma virus (HPV), transmitted during sexual intercourse, has been implicated in the induction of cervical cancer.

- Genital warts are the visible manifestations of the presence of the HPV, but the virus may also exist invisibly in the genital tract.

- Predisposing factors to cervical cancer include sex, age of first intercourse, smoking, lower social class, poverty, occupation, narcotics, and genetics.

- Certain aspects of sexual behaviour of both men and women, such as promiscuity, influence the risk of developing cervical cancer.

- Most cervical cancers are of the squamous cell variety and occur only in non-virginal women. However, up to 10 per cent of cervical cancers are adenocarcinomas which develop in the columnar epithelium and occur in both virginal and non-virginal women.

Where and what is the cervix?

The cervix is a round, firm, mushroom-like structure which joins the uterus to the vagina. In its centre, the cervix has an opening, called the external os (os = mouth), which leads to a narrow canal called the cervical canal. This canal leads into and opens through the internal os into the uterus. These passages and openings allow for menstrual discharge to pass from the uterus through the canal and cervix into the vagina and then to the outside during a woman's period. Glands within the linings of the cervix and vagina produce a variety of secretions which have several important functions.

The cervix plays a significant role in human reproduction. It is at the centre of the female reproductive organs and of the reproductive system. As well as allowing the outward flow of discharges and secretions, the os is the gateway through which sperm

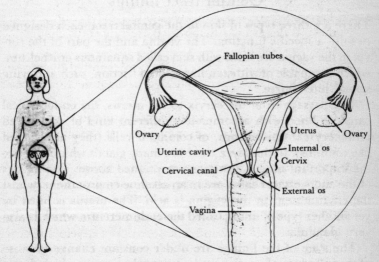

Figure 1 The female reproductive organs.

enter the cervical canal and eventually gain access to the ovum. Sperm entry, travel and fertilization are facilitated by mucus-producing glands (*Endocervical* glands) within the cervix, and this mucus lubricates the vagina during sexual intercourse. During pregnancy the cervix holds the baby in the uterus and it opens during delivery.

What is cervical cancer?

Cervical cancer begins as *pre-cancer* on and in the cells of the skin lining the cervix. These pre-cancerous cells show characteristic changes which suggest a potential to become cancerous, a situation where the cells multiply uncontrollably and form tumours (cancerous masses) which grow into and beyond the cervix. Furthermore, cancerous cells may metastasize i.e. they break off from such tumours and pass to other parts of the body where they can lodge and form other tumours. To understand how and where cervical cancer develops, it is necessary to appreciate the structure and function of the female genital tract.

Genital tract linings

There are three types of skin in the genital tract, each designed to fulfil a specific function. The vagina and the part of the cervix in the vagina are lined with skin called **squamous epithelium**, which is capable of withstanding a lot of friction, such as during sexual intercourse.

The passage from the cervix to the uterus, the endocervical canal, is lined with a completely different kind of skin called **endocervical epithelium**, of columnar cells (they are shaped like columns). In this layer, there are many glands which produce the important mucus secretions mentioned above. The linings of the endocervical canal are in an alkaline environment, whilst the environment in the vagina is acid. The uterus is lined by yet another type of lining called the **endometrium** which is also very glandular.

The state of the linings are under constant change because of the influence of ovarian and pituitary hormones which determine their thickness, secretion of fluids, and cell growth.

Squamocolumnar junction

The point at which the two different types of skin lining the vagina and cervix meet is called the **squamocolumnar junction** (SCJ). It is here that the initial cancerous changes (pre-cancer) which may ultimately lead to cervical cancer begin. Before puberty, and after the menopause, that junction is situated inside the endocervical canal at a small distance from the external cervical os.

Transformation zone

During puberty and adolescence, more oestrogen is produced which increases the thickness and amounts of all the linings in the genital tract. As a result of this, the original squamocolumnar junction situated inside the endocervical canal migrates down and everts out into the vagina from its original position before puberty in the endocervical canal and appears on the vaginal part of the cervix. The area on the cervix which is now covered by this migrated columnar epithelium from the cervical canal is called the **transformation zone**. The columnar epithelium has thus changed its environment from alkaline (inside the cervical canal) to acid (in the vagina). The acid fluid in the vagina tends to break down the migrated columnar epithelium. Such an area may appear raw (reddish in colour) to the naked eye and is often described as an **erosion**. Meanwhile, the squamous epithelium (which lines the vagina and part of the cervix) begins to grow from beneath the columnar epithelium and gradually replaces it. This normal replacement of one type of lining by another is called squamous metaplasia (meta = half, plasia = formation).

In time, **squamous metaplasia** is complete and irreversible. The change is gradual, taking several years during and after puberty. A new skin may cover the entire transformation zone, and the process is well underway by the time a woman is in her late teens. After the menopause the reverse process takes place, the ovarian hormones diminish, the epithelium shrinks and the transformation zone together with the squamocolumnar junction are drawn back up high into the canal.

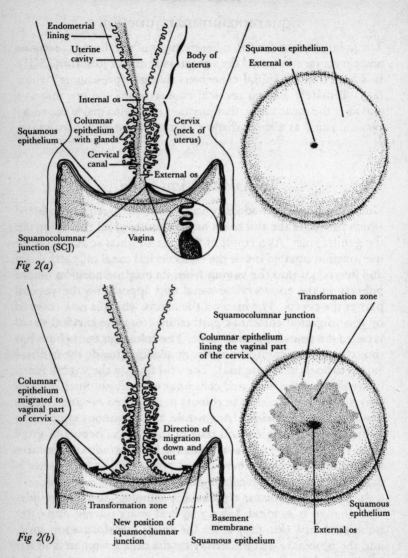

Figure 2 a) The position of the genital linings in pre-puberty. The figure on the right shows the surface of the cervix, the figure on the left shows the cervix in cross-section. b) The adolescent cervix. The area covered by the migrated columnar epithelium is called the transformation zone,

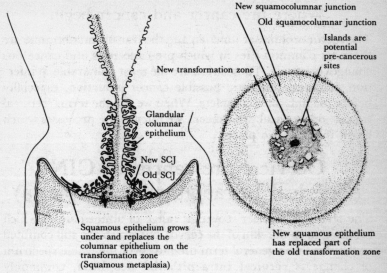

New squamocolumnar junction

Old squamocolumnar junction

Islands are potential pre-cancerous sites

New transformation zone

Glandular columnar epithelium

New SCJ
Old SCJ

Squamous epithelium grows under and replaces the columnar epithelium on the transformation zone (Squamous metaplasia)

New squamous epithelium has replaced part of the old transformation zone

Fig 2(c)

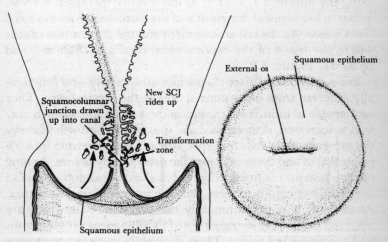

Squamous epithelium

External os

New SCJ rides up

Squamocolumnar junction drawn up into canal

Transformation zone

Squamous epithelium

Fig 2(d)

and is the prime site of pre-cancerous changes. c) The post-adolescent cervix. d) The post-menopausal cervix. The transformation zone has now been drawn up into the cervical canal.

Where pre-cancer and cancer begin

The squamocolumnar junction and the transformation zone are the most common sites at which pre-cancerous and cancerous changes originate. These areas are the most vulnerable to infection, inflammation, and possible cancer induction, especially before metaplasia is complete. When we use the terms 'cervical cancer' or 'cervical pre-cancer', we refer to the processes which begin in these two places.

Cervical pre-cancer or CIN (Cervical Intraepithelial Neoplasia)

The term 'pre-cancer' covers a range of abnormalities which occur on or in the skin of the cervix, but which are still confined in the skin. The general term used to cover the whole spectrum of change is **cervical intraepithelial neoplasia**, commonly abbreviated to CIN. The degree of abnormality is specified by using the numbers 1, 2, or 3, as the severity increases. CIN is, in fact, a histological description of the disturbance within a cell (see Chapter 4), the cell arrangement and the distribution of cells within the tissue of the cervical skin. (See p.51, Figure 5 and pp.82-83, Figure 8.)

Pre-cancerous cells are chemically, structurally, and functionally different from other normal cells in the cervical skin. They are capable of inducing a change in their neighbours which may lead to increased, disorganized and uncontrolled growth whereby the pre-cancerous cells multiply, spread, and penetrate into the cervical skin and eventually into the deeper body tissues. As long as they remain confined to the cervical skin and do not spread beyond these confines, these cells are described as *pre-cancerous*. At present, it is predominantly the nuclei of cells which are observed as showing changes related to subsequent pre-cancerous and cancerous behaviour. These changes in nuclear appearance are described as mild, moderate, or severe dyskaryosis (disturbance of the nucleus). Mild dyskaryotic (pre-cancerous) changes may be reversible and do not necessarily progress to cancer. Moderate or severely dyskaryotic cells are likely to go beyond the point of no return, and if they are not removed, they become cancerous.

However, the complete removal of all pre-cancerous cells, whatever their degree of dyskaryosis, should halt the progression to the cancerous state and penetration (invasion) beyond the cervical skin.

How cervical cancer develops

A cancerous situation is one where cells have advanced from a pre-cancerous state into one where they grow uncontrollably. They grow into, penetrate, and invade the surrounding underlying tissues and form malignant tumours (balls of cancerous cells). These cells may break off and spread (metastasize) via the lymphatic channels and the blood vessels to other organs in the body where they may lodge and similarly multiply uncontrollably into tumours. These tumours harm the body by compressing vital structures in organs at the expense of their normal function, leading to deterioration of health and, ultimately, to death if not treated.

In the case of cervical cancer, once a tumour begins to form, it grows deeper and deeper into the cervix. Eventually it grows into the body of the uterus, into the vagina, rectum, bowel and bladder. It can enter and spread into the lymphatic channels and lymph nodes. These nodes have a vital role to play in the body's defence system. They produce **lymphocytes**, special cells capable of destroying infective organisms. These lymphocytes also fight cancer cells, halting their growth and spread. The significance of cancer cells in entering the lymphatic system is that they are carried along lymphatic channels into the lymph glands where they lodge, multiply, and enlarge the gland from where they may also break off and be carried along the lymphatic channels into the blood stream.

Once they have entered the blood stream in this way, cancer cells can circulate around the body and lodge in various organs where they grow and multiply. The way in which cancer is spread around the body from an initial site of cancer is known as *metastasis*.

The development from a pre-cancerous to a cancerous condition is like a spot of rust on a car door, which, if not put right quickly, will spread and destroy the door and, eventually, the entire car body. The speed with which the pre-cancerous state develops into cancer and subsequently becomes invasive and spreads, varies between individuals and there are at present no tests which enable the rate of progression to be predicted accurately. It can take as long as ten years or as short a time as one year for pre-cancer to develop into cancer.

Cervical adenocarcinoma

This book deals specifically with a form of cervical cancer technically known as **squamous cell carcinoma** of the cervix which occurs in the squamous epithelium of the squamocolumnar junction of transformation zone of the cervix. Although the vast majority (90 to 98 per cent) of carcinomas of the cervix are squamous cell carcinomas, up to 10 per cent of cervical cancers are of a type known as **adenocarcinoma**. This type of cervical cancer occurs in the glands of the columnar epithelium, present in the recesses and folds deep in the endocervical canal. This form of cancer is harder to detect than squamous cell abnormalities simply because it is beyond the reach of the standard techniques used to sample cells from the cervix (the cervical smear). Recent evidence has shown that this type of cancer may exist in virginal women.

What causes cervical cancer?

The fact that squamous cell carcinoma type does not occur in virginal women clearly suggests that this type of cancer may be considered to be a sexually transmitted disease, or at least a disease whose onset is somehow related to sex.

Over the last thirty years many factors have been considered and continue to be scrutinized as possible causal agents. In addition to semen itself, a wide variety of bacterial and viral infections are individually or jointly suspected of initiating this change in the cervix. The cervix itself may form a favourable area in which the pre-cancerous change is either induced or propagated and in which many genetic, immunological, hormonal, and environmental factors are suspected of playing a part in the progression or regression of this change.

The most likely infective agent now seems to be the human papilloma virus (HPV) which is found in the cells of the genital tract and rectum of both men and women. There are nearly fifty varieties of HPV, each of which is denoted by a number. It is possible to distinguish between these varieties by using the latest diagnostic techniques in biotechnology. This virus, known commonly as the wart virus, can exist in cells without any signs or symptoms, but may manifest itself in the form of genital warts which are visible to the naked eye. The virus is thought to be transmitted from an infected to a non-infected sexual partner during intercourse and its presence can be identified by taking samples from the genital tract and analysing them using a method of comparing DNA from samples with reference genetic material. (DNA is an essential component within the cell nucleus and carries the genetic coding which dictates development and eventual tissue characteristics.)

The damaged cervical cells show certain changes which can be seen under a microscope. The cell nucleus appears bigger with a darker nuclear material and cytoplasm (the area between the nucleus and the cell membrane) forming a sort of halo around the nucleus. Cells affected in this way are called **koilocytes**.

The presence of koilocytes on microscopic observation suggests infection with a virus, and it has been shown that in many pre-cancerous states associated with the presence of the virus, the pre-cancer sooner or later progresses to a fully cancerous condition.

It has become increasingly evident that genital warts in men and women are associated with a higher incidence of cervical cancer, and it is suspected that cervical cancer may be induced by the human papilloma virus. In a study at the Royal Northern Hospital (M.J. Campion *et al.*, *Lancet* 1986, *2*, p.237) of 100 women with CIN 1, 39 per cent of them had evidence of HPV 16 infection. Of the women whose CIN 1 progressed to the more severe CIN 3, the detection rate was 85 per cent. The authors concluded that the detection of HPV 16 appears to identify women at high risk of rapid progression from CIN 1 to CIN 3 and that they should be treated promptly.

The HPV types that seem to be associated with pre-cancers of the genital areas include human papilloma viruses 6, 11, 16, and 18. HPV 16 recovered from pre-cancerous tissues has been found in around 70-80 per cent of cases of CIN 3s and carcinomas *in situ*, as well as in cancerous tissues. The virus particles are incorporated in the DNA of the host cell's nuclei and this particular wart virus has been detected in cancer cells.

Where HPV has been identified in as yet mildly pre-cancerous cells, these cells have a high chance of progressing to malignancy. In the study of women referred to above, 26 per cent of early pre-cancers (CIN 1) progressed to histologically proven CIN 3 within two years, but only 7 per cent regressed to normal.

It is known that HPV is found in the female genital tract, but if this virus is to be considered a cancer-causing agent, it is necessary to know when and how HPV is involved in the cancerous process, and whether its presence is essential for cancerous changes to occur.

Evidence that HPV is associated with cervical cancer has come from many worldwide sources including that of virologist Dennis McCance and gynaecologist Albert Singer of the Royal Northern Hospital in London. However, it is not yet certain whether this is a chance association. It could be that the action of the virus is not one of direct induction of pre-cancer and cancer of the cervix, but may be triggered by the presence of other factors. It may also be possible that the wart virus assists or is assisted by yet another agent to cause pre-cancer. A lot more research needs to be done before the agent or agents which induce cervical pre-cancers and cancers are indisputably identified.

Predisposing factors to cervical cancer

The covering epithelium on the surface of the cervix is a type of skin which is susceptible to cancer. It has recently been reported that there has been an overall increase in all types of skin cancers in many parts of the world. It is interesting to conjecture whether this is associated with alteration in diet, vitamin or mineral deficiencies or a change in the ozone layer. However, there are a number of well-identified risk factors which seem to predispose women to cervical cancer.

Sex

Since the mid-19th century there have been many studies linking the risk of cervical cancer with the sexual behaviours of both men and women. One of the most important factors to consider is the age at which a woman first has intercourse.

The younger a woman has intercourse, the greater the risk of developing cervical cancer. Some statistics indicate that having intercourse before the age of 21 poses the greatest risk. For example, a joint study by the Imperial Cancer Research Fund, the University of Oxford, and the John Radcliffe Infirmary in Oxford (R.W.C. Harris *et al.*, *British Journal of Cancer* 1980, *42*, p.359), showed that the relative risk of pre-cancer was higher the younger the age of first intercourse (see Table 2 for comparison of risks). 237 women who attended the John Radcliffe and Churchill Hospitals in Oxford with abnormal cervical smears were analysed in the study. Cervical biopsies taken from the women were classified as carcinoma *in situ* (65 women), severe dysplasia (81), mild dysplasia (44) and normal histology (47). (Biopsy results are classified in terms of CIN but smears are described in terms of dyskaryosis).

Table 2 **Relative risks of cervical abnormalities according to age of first intercourse**

Age at first intercourse (years)	Normal histology	Mild dysplasia	Severe dysplasia	Carcinoma *in situ*
21 + or never	1.00	1.00	1.00	1.00
19-20	1.56	1.29	1.45	1.11
17-18	1.76	1.91	1.85	3.41
<17	0.62	3.33	2.94	1.69

It was also shown in the study that the risk of cervical abnormalities increased with the number of sexual partners. In all four groups shown in Table 3, the risk was higher among women who had had two partners than those who had had one, and higher still among women who had had three or more partners.

Table 3 **Relative risk of cervical abnormalities according to number of sexual partners**

Number of sexual partners	Normal histology	Mild dysplasia	Severe dysplasia	Carcinoma *in situ*
0-1	1.00	1.00	1.00	1.00
2	2.49	1.11	2.67	5.21
3-5	7.01	3.96	8.49	7.92
6 +	0.63	10.74	16.79	14.20

However, when the data from Table 2 and Table 3 was compared (see Table 4), the result showed that although there was an increase across each age group in the relative risk of cervical abnormalities with increased number of sexual partners, there was no clear relationship of risk at age of first intercourse when the number of sexual partners was taken into account. In other words, the younger a woman begins to have sex, the larger the number of partners she is likely to have, and it is this which is the over-riding influence on the likelihood of cervical cancer developing. It used to be thought that increased vulnerability of the cervix during metaplasia was responsible for an increased risk of developing a cervical abnormality. However, it now seems that there is a stronger connection with the number of sexual partners, which indicates it is the number of partners that is the important factor, suggesting that cervical cancer is a sexually transmitted disease.

The risk also rises for women whose husbands begin intercourse at an early age. In another study at the John Radcliffe and Churchill Hospitals in Oxford, (J.D. Buckley *et al.*, *Lancet*, 1981, **2**, p.1010), researchers interviewed husbands of 31 women with cervical abnormalities (cancer or pre-cancer) who had had no other partner other than their husband. The aim was to deter-

Table 4 Relative risks of cervical abnormalities according to age of first intercourse and number of sexual partners

Age at first intercourse (years)	Number of sexual partners			
	0-1	2	3-5	6+
21 + or never	1.00	2.42	7.09	6.44
19-20	0.81	1.93	15.04	12.89
17-18	1.40	5.09	5.98	10.03
<17	1.55	1.90	8.82	7.52

Source: [tables 2, 3, 4]: R.W.C. Harris *et al.*, *British Journal of Cancer*, volume 42, p.359, 1980.

mine whether cervical abnormalities in women could be related to their husband's sexual background.

Table 5 shows that the more sexual partners the husband has had, the greater the relative risk of a cervical abnormality in their current partner. Similarly, the earlier the age of first intercourse of the husband, the greater the likelihood that the wife will con-

Table 5 Relative risks of cervical abnormalities according to selected characteristics of the husbands

	Dysplasia and carcinoma *in situ*	Invasive carcinoma	Combined relative risk
No. of sexual partners			
1	1.00	1.00	1.00
2-5	2.13	1.20	1.65
6-15	2.74	2.42	2.63
16 or more	9.84	6.76	7.82
Age at first intercourse			
Over 21	1.00	1.00	1.00
19-20	6.18	1.99	3.10
17-18	7.05	2.44	3.96
<17	8.05	2.78	4.22

tract a cervical abnormality. The figures in Table 5 add weight to the idea that cervical abnormalities are sexually transmitted. One might also conclude that men who have had sex with women who have cervical abnormalities are more likely to pick up and transmit cancer-inducing agents to their next partner. However, one need not be very promiscuous to acquire the disease. It may take only one act of sexual intercourse to become affected.

Men who have genital warts are more likely to infect their female partners with genital warts. The viruses which cause these warts may subsequently be involved in causing pre-cancer and eventually cancer on the cervix and occasionally elsewhere in the vaginal and vulval area. A study by doctors at the Royal Northern, Whittington and Guy's Hospitals, showed that there was an increased risk of CIN in women whose male partners had penile warts (M.J. Campion *et al.*, *Lancet*, 1985, **1**, p.943.) 76 per cent of the women had, or had recently had, symptoms of HPV infection, and 36 per cent had CIN.

Another study by Dr Thomas Allerding and his colleagues from the University of New Mexico School of Medicine showed that koilocytes, indicating the presence of human papilloma virus, were found in 25 per cent of 67 women who had carcinoma *in situ* or invasive cancer (T.J Allerding *et al.*, *Acta Cytologica*, 1985 **29**, 5, p.655). They also found presence of infection by the micro-organism *Chlamydia trachomatis* in 27 per cent of the women. The bacteria causes an inflammatory response and inflammation often accompanies or may be the result of pre-cancer. Much more research needs to be done on the inflammatory response in cervical tissue before linking other agents with pre-cancerous change.

Research at the Hammersmith Hospital in London has shown that frequent exposure of the cervix to chemicals in semen may lower its immunological defences against cancer. Other researchers have shown this effect to be enhanced by exposure to semen from a number of partners.

Age at first pregnancy and number of pregnancies

There is conflicting evidence as to whether an early first pregnancy (younger than 20) or a large number of pregnancies puts women at greater risk of cervical cancer.

Smoking

Several studies have indicated that cigarette smoking by either partner is a major risk factor in developing cervical cancer. The risk further increases when both partners smoke. The Third National Cancer Survey in 1977, discovered a strong correlation between smoking and cervical cancer. It was suggested that this correlation is a reflection of other sexual or social behaviour, but even when these were accounted for, smoking still turned out to be a significant risk factor. The reason for this is not yet clear, but as cervical tissue has the ability to extract and concentrate various substances from the blood, it may be that cancer-causing agents in tobacco are concentrated in the cervix, where they exert a variety of changes. These may exacerbate the effects of a cancer-causing agent such as a virus, or simply make the cervix more susceptible to change, and these could act as a cancerous complement to viral infection. It is also possible that smokers have a lowered immune system. For instance, research at the Royal Northern and Whittington Hospitals has shown that in smokers there is a significant decrease in the Langerhans cell population as compared to non-smokers (S.E Barton *et al.*, *Lancet*, ii, p.652, 1988). The lack of such cells is thought to reduce the cervix's immunological defence mechanisms, which may ultimately be shown to lead to susceptibility to infection and subsequent cancerous change.

Contraceptives

It is debatable whether the use of the contraceptive pill is linked to an increased risk of cervical cancer. A 1983 report of a study by the Family Planning Association and Professor Martin Vessey and others at Oxford University, suggested the Pill was linked to an increased rate of pre-cancerous change which was shown to be more than twice as high in women who had been on the Pill for eight years than those who used an IUD (an intrauterine device also known as a coil).

In his book on contraception, Dr John Guillebaud, medical director of the Margaret Pyke Centre in London, suggests that the balance of evidence supports the idea that the Pill *may* act as a *weak* co-factor in inducing a pre-cancerous change if it is used long term. However, he points out that there is no evidence that the Pill itself is a carcinogen and its influence is clearly much less than the influence of sexual lifestyle.

The exclusive use of barrier methods of contraception such as the cap or the condom is associated with lower incidence of the disease possibly because they prevent the semen, bacterial and viral carcinogens from reaching the cervix.

Occupation and social class

One of the most significant risk factors is poverty. Cervical cancer is most likely to kill Puerto Ricans, deprived blacks and poor whites in the United States, and is the major cancer killer of women in the developing world. In Britain, mortality statistics show it to have the steepest social-class gradient of any cancer. This can be explained in two ways. Firstly, illegitimate births and abortions are more frequent among the lower classes and this may reflect increased sexual activity. The second factor is that each class is associated with certain types of occupation which in itself is associated with a particular risk of acquiring cervical cancer. It is the occupation of the male partner which is most relevant here.

Table 6 shows the relative degree of risk from certain occupations and in which social class they are found. Clearly the risk is greater in those occupations in the lower social classes. The male occupations which are associated with an increased risk of cervical cancer in women include manual labour where men may face poor or unhygienic work conditions and are themselves more likely to suffer from cancers of the genital region or lung. Women working in the textile industry are at higher risk, supposedly from their exposure to oily textile wastes which may be transmitted from the hand to the genital region or may be absorbed through the skin into the body and concentrate in the cervix.

Table 6 **Mortality rates in married women for cervical cancer by social class and husbands' occupation (England and Wales 1959-63)**

Social class	Occupations of husband	*SMR
I	**All occupations** (average)	34
	Clergymen	12
	Scientists	17
	Civil engineers	60
II	**All occupations** (average)	64
	Senior government officials	40
	Teachers	30
	Publicans and inn keepers	120
	Hotel and boarding house keepers	150
III	**All occupations** (average)	100
	Crane and hoist operators	159
	Clerks of works	50
	Clerks	64
	Drivers of road goods vehicles	168
IV	**All occupations** (average)	116
	Shopkeepers and assistants	71
	Gardeners and groundsmen	98
	Fishermen	257
	Deck and engine room ratings, barge and boatmen	263
V	**All occupations** (average)	181
	Office and window cleaners	95
	Labourers	222

Source: Registrar General's occupational mortality tables for England and Wales.
*SMR: Standardized Mortality Ratio

Genetics

There is evidence to suggest that there may be a genetic influence in the risk of cervical cancer developing. It may be that some women have a reduced immunity of their cervical skin to the biological damage it suffers from the effects of or agents carried

by sperm. Such damage includes sperm breakdown products and enzymes (chemicals important in controlling the body's metabolism) which are released from the degeneration of blood cells and bacteria and viruses on the cervical skin.

Now it seems that there may exist a protective agent in the cervical epithelium and mucus, known as alpha-antitrypsin, which is able to neutralize these enzymes and other biological breakdown products. The blood levels of this protective agent are controlled by a well-defined genetic system and in some women there are genes which code for decreased synthesis and the presence of such genes seems to be correlated with the development of cervical cancer.

Drugs

There is a wide variety of drugs especially designed to lower one's natural immunity. These immuno-suppressive drugs are used in transplant surgery and in suppression of auto-immune diseases such as ulcerative colitis, thyroid disorders and rheumatoid arthritis. As many viruses are now regarded as causing pre-cancer and cancer, a woman whose immunity has been compromised by these drugs is therefore at increased risk of cervical cancer. Female smokers and heroin addicts must regard themselves as being at a significantly greater risk of cervical cancer as heroin and tobacco have similar effects in reducing immunity.

In order to find out more about any abnormalities on the cervix, your GP or clinic may recommended a number of further tests, which are described in the next chapter.

Chapter 3

Detecting cervical cancer — the cervical smear

- Cervical cancer can exist in a woman long before it gives rise to any signs or symptoms.
- The cervical smear is the chief method of detecting cervical abnormalities such as pre-cancerous and cancerous change and is 70-90 per cent accurate.
- Early detection gives an opportunity for early effective treatment.
- 60-90 per cent of women who die of cervical cancer have never had a smear.
- Pelvic examination at the time of screening by cervical smears affords additional screening for other possible pelvic abnormalities, e.g. ovarian or uterine cancers and pelvic infections.
- The frequency of smears needed to safeguard against the disease depends on individual characteristics and these include: sexual behaviour of oneself and one's partner; presence of genital warts on either partner; previous history of abnormal smears or CIN.
- The degree of pre-cancerous abnormalities in cervical smears are described as mild, moderate, or severe dyskaryosis which refers to the nuclear disturbance in the cell.
- There are many inherent errors in the system of analysis and reporting of smears. You should check your result if it fails to arrive.

The modern detection of cervical cancer owes much to a medically qualified Greek zoologist called George Nicholaus Papanicolaou (1889-1962) who lived in the United States at the turn of this century, and is regarded as the father of modern cytology (the study of cells). Through his study of vaginal and cervical cells he showed that there were cyclical changes in the shape and size of the nucleus in the cell and also changes in the way they reacted to and were stained by the various dyes he used. He deduced that cell alterations were both caused by and reflected the changing hormonal levels and other constituents in the blood.

It became apparent that there existed a wide spectrum of cellular abnormalities, some of which disappeared, while some progressed into pre-cancerous and then cancerous states.

In 1925 Papanicolaou wrote and published his first paper which he presented at a conference in Battlecreek, Michigan in 1928 in which he stated:

> In carcinoma (cancer) of the cervix, cancer cells are usually present in smears. These can be identified even more easily than infections because they are isolated and show certain morphological (shape) changes. Certain cases of carcinoma of the cervix may be diagnosed by the presence of only one of these cells.

In 1941, he and Herbert Traut presented another paper to the New York Obstetric Society. Dr Isador Rubin of Mount Sinai hospital said:

> If this vaginal smear proves diagnostic in a large number of cases of the hidden type of carcinoma and of the early hitherto unrecognizable carcinoma of the cervix by the usual means at our disposal, including the colposcope, then we have made a great advance in the diagnostic armamentarium in this field.

However, it is only now that the medical profession understands the importance of pre-symptomatic detection using smears, the need for the training of pathologists and cytologists, and the necessity of persuading women to understand the importance of detection of the disease by means of cervical smears.

It is now widely accepted that examination of cervical smears will detect the presence of abnormal cervical cells and treatment can be carried out at an early stage before the disease has developed and invaded to a degree where it threatens a woman's fertility and even her life.

In 1943 Papanicolaou showed that cervical cancer could be detected in women who did not have the symptoms of cervical cancer, not just those who had a clearly definable cancer, and Papanicolaou and Traut introduced the 'Pap smear' as a method of early detection of carcinoma of the cervix. After the Second World War, screening women by taking cervical smears from gynaecological patients started in various countries throughout the world. One of the earliest programmes was in British Columbia where screening was initiated in 1947. In Britain, cervical smear testing was started in the 1950s. The taking of cervical smears from gynaecological patients was initiated in the North-East of Scotland in 1958. In 1960 Professor Sir Dugald Baird, an obstetrician and gynaecologist who pioneered cervical screening in Scotland, suggested that *all* women should have the opportunity to have this test. At this stage, it was not known who should be screened or when and how often this should be done. Indeed, these aspects are still a subject of dispute and change. However, it is now recognized by the whole medical profession that the key to detection of cervical cancer is having cervical smears.

The cervical smear

A cervical smear is the collection of cells from the cervix and vagina. Abnormalities in these cells can be detected in the laboratory with the aid of a microscope. This test is currently the chief screening technique used in the identification of cervical precancer.

Cells from adenocarcinomas (the rarer type of cervical cancer which exists in the folds and ridges of the endocervical epithelium) occasionally appear on the slide. The importance of this particular form of carcinoma of the cervix is that unless identification is made, this cancer will progress in very much the same way as the squamous cell carcinoma and may ultimately prove fatal. Early identification allows for early, and usually completely successful treatment in which all pre-cancerous cells are simply and completely removed which prevents the development of pre-cancer to cancer. Yet, the vast majority of women (between 60 and 90 per cent) who die of cervical cancer have never had a cervical smear.

Who should have a cervical smear?

All women should have a cervical smear. The first smear should be within a year of a woman first having sex and smears should continue until the age of 70. This group includes even the very young, as research has shown that sexually active teenage girls, even those under the age of 16, are prone to develop cervical pre-cancer. (See also p.48 on frequency of smears.)

Smears can stop if a woman has had three consecutive smears leading up to her 70th birthday and she no longer has sexual intercourse. Women over the age of 70 who are still sexually active should continue to have regular smears.

Screening virginal women

Although squamous cell carcinoma is found only in women who have had sexual intercourse, there is a possibility of detecting an adenocarcinoma present in both virginal and non-virginal women. Regular screening is recommended for virginal women at the same frequency as for non-virginal women, but it is worth noting that most adenocarcinomas occur after the age of 25, and most of these are found in women between the ages of 60 and 70. Although virginal women may not wish to have a smear, it is vital that they do so if they experience any unusual bleeding or discharge from the vagina, as this may be the hallmark of a genital cancer (cervix, uterus, or Fallopian tubes). All post-menopausal bleeding must be similarly investigated.

Why have a cervical smear?

If abnormal pre-cancerous or cancerous cells are detected early enough, long before the disease gives rise to any signs or symptoms, it is possible to destroy the abnormal cells completely by removing all the affected skin using one of the methods described in Chapter 5. By doing so, it is possible to save lives and prevent damage to organs involved in sex and reproduction, such as the uterus and cervix, and to save the patient from a major operation such as a hysterectomy (removal of the cervix and uterus) which is necessary when the disease is more advanced.

Cervical screening is the chief method of detection of cervical cancer, and it is a simple procedure. If a cervical abnormality is suspected it is necessary to investigate it further by a technique known as colposcopy (which will be discussed in detail in Chapter 4) before any treatment is chosen.

Where are cervical smears taken?

There are a number of places and situations in which a woman may be offered a cervical smear. These may be during gynaecological or family planning appointments, obstetric or antenatal check-ups, well-woman check-ups, opportunist smears during examinations for unconnected medical conditions, and organized call and recall appointments specifically for cervical smears. Women may be visited at home, particularly those in social class 4 and 5, to provide smears.

Such smears should be carried out by medical and nursing practitioners who should be well trained in the technique of taking smears. This may take place in general practitioner surgeries, health centres which include cervical screening, companies who have their employees screened on site, and special centres organized for this purpose such as clinics or travelling caravans.

What is involved in attending for a cervical smear?

When booking an appointment to have a smear, which should normally be done in advance, women should try to ensure it does not coincide with the expected date of a period as this may result in the smear being obscured by blood. Similarly, and ideally, condoms should be used for the few days prior to a smear to ensure the slide will not be obscured by semen. If a vaginal cap is used with contraceptive cream within 24 hours of a smear, the cream may similarly obscure the cells on the slide. If a woman is suffering from a vaginal discharge caused by an infection, the infection should be treated before a smear is taken.

When attending for a smear, a woman will be asked for the following information: full surname and forename, date of birth, address and telephone number for smear results to be sent, details of any possible change of address in the near future, name and address of the family doctor, date of the first day of the last menstrual period, number of pregnancies (miscarriage and abortions included), if she uses contraception and, if so, what form, hormonal treatment other than for contraception, past or present gynaecological abnormalities and subsequent treatments, dates and results of previous cervical smears, details of unusual intermenstrual, post-coital, or post-menopausal bleeding; occupation (one's own and/or one's sexual partner(s)).

Women should ask: When the results are likely to be ready, how they will be communicated to them, and to whom and where to enquire in case the results fail to be notified. The last point is particularly important as some centres will only notify women if the result is abnormal. This is not a very safe system because, for a variety of reasons, an abnormal result may not be conveyed to a patient.

What happens when a smear is taken?

Before having a smear it is important to empty one's bladder. This will make the process and any examination more comfortable. Underclothes are removed and the woman is asked to lie on her back on an examination couch. To help with the examination she needs to bend her knees and open her legs well apart. At this stage the doctor or nurse can inspect the whole genital area and check for any abnormalities such as warts, rashes, spots, or discharge.

Just before, or sometimes after, the smear is taken, there should be a gentle pelvic examination. For hygienic reasons, the doctor or nurse puts a thin plastic glove on to the examining hand. Two fingers (index and middle finger) are gently inserted into the vagina, whilst the other hand is placed over the abdomen. This examination enables the size, shape, and position of the uterus, tubes and ovaries to be determined. It can help identify abnormalities such as uterine fibroids, ovarian cysts, tubal masses, and pelvic inflammatory disease. Failure to perform such an examination when a woman is attending for a smear may mean abnormalities are not detected.

If a male doctor or nurse performs the gynaecological examination, it is customary to have a female member of staff present to chaperone the doctor. Unfortunately, not all screening centres have personnel adequately trained and skilled in performing such an examination and in such cases only a cervical smear may be taken. Some centres may have a policy to offer a full medical examination, including blood pressure, urine analysis, breast examination, and contraceptive check-up where possible.

Once the position of the cervix has been ascertained, a warmed closed metal instrument called a vaginal speculum is inserted gently and painlessly into the vagina. It is then gently opened to part the vaginal walls and allow access to the cervix which is high up inside the vagina. The cervix and vagina may then be visually inspected and if there is any evidence of discharge or a history of one, a swab of the area may be taken with a cotton wool-tipped wooden, sterile applicator. This type of sampling is known as a High Vaginal Swab (HVS) and should not be confused with a cervical smear. The swab is placed in a small container filled with a special fluid which keeps the bacteria alive, and sent the same day to a laboratory for investigation for the presence of an infection. If there is a profuse discharge, it may have to be wiped away gently in order to reveal the surface of the cervix and enable adequate inspection.

The next step involves sweeping the entire surface of the cervix, including part of the cervical canal, with a specially shaped spatula. Occasionally, in addition to using the spatula, a small brush called a cytobrush may be used to collect cells from inside the cervical canal. The material collected by the spatula and cytobrush should contain cells from the vagina, cervix, and endocervical canal. This must be spread on to a glass slide immediately which should have previously been labelled with the patient's name, date of birth, and date of test. The slide is flooded immediately with a special fixing solution which sticks and preserves the cells on the slide which can then be transported to the laboratory. There, the cells are stained with various diag-

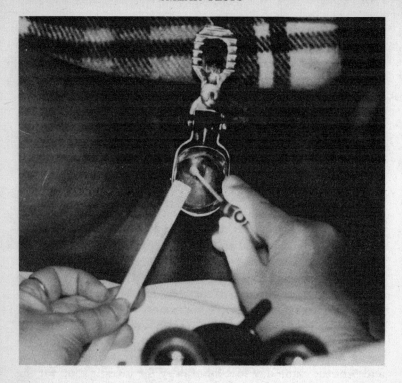

Figure 3 Taking a High Vaginal Swab.

nostic dyes and examined and reported on. Such slides can be kept for future reference for years to come.

As soon as the smear has been collected, the speculum is removed from the vagina and the woman is asked to dress. Sometimes a slight blood-stained discharge is noticed soon after the smear was taken. This is usually due to the cervix bleeding slightly which may happen after it has been scraped by the spatula and is perfectly normal and nothing to worry about.

The final check

Immediately after the test and before the woman leaves, a final check should be made to ensure that all observations have been

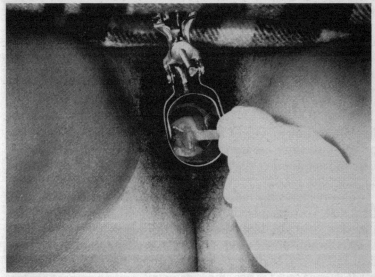

Fig 4(a)

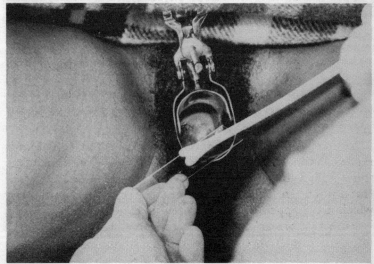

Fig 4(b)

Figure 4 a) Taking a cervical smear. b) Spreading the sample.

written down, documentation completed, correct addresses for communication verified, and any expected change of address noted down. The taking of the smear takes just a few minutes, and with undressing, dressing and discussion with the medical staff, the whole process should be over in around fifteen minutes.

Problems in getting a smear taken

Not all doctors or nurses have the necessary training, facilities or administrative set-up to take smears. It may then be necessary to visit another doctor, family planning centre or hospital to have one taken.

Some doctors may refuse to give smears at a greater frequency than that recommended by Government guidelines and for which they are paid. In 1990 the guidelines instructed GPs to take smears from women aged 25 to 64 every five years. An 80 per cent uptake by eligible patients qualified the GP for full payment, 50 per cent for two thirds payment, and no payment below a 50 per cent uptake. Excluded from payments are smears taken from women outside the 25-64 age group, or those who need additional or repeat smears, or who are not on the GP's register. Women who want more regular smears must hope that whichever centre they approach will be prepared to provide them. Alternatively, a woman can go to a private clinic for a smear. However, some doctors would prefer to see a maximum three year interval between smears (and a yearly interval for women who have been treated for a pre-cancer or cancer).

Who is most likely to have a smear?

- Well-informed women who present themselves for a test at self-initiated and regular intervals. Such women are often middle or upper class.

- Women who attend family planning or antenatal clinics and are offered opportunist screening.

- Women who respond to a call or recall from a doctor, or health authority in conjunction with local or national guidelines for repeat-smearing, or whose employers organize such screening.

Who is likely to miss having a smear?

- Women who do not know about the disease.

- Women who know about the disease but are under the impression that they are not prone to contracting it. This includes many married women, those in stable relationships, older and post-menopausal women, and virginal women.

- Women who know about the disease but would prefer not to know whether they have it or not. This is often caused by sheer fear of the disease.

- Women who do not use any methods of contraception or who obtain contraceptives over the counter. These women are not regular attenders at the doctor's surgery, local health centre or family planning clinic where screening may be carried out. This group may also include long-term cap users, lesbians, women who have been sterilized, and post-menopausal women.

- Women who are afraid of a smear because they think it may be painful.

- Women who are reluctant to have a smear because of potential embarrassment. As doctors see naked patients every day there is nothing to be shy about.

- Women who do not receive a call or recall notice either because such a system does not exist in their area or because they cannot be traced if they have moved.

- Women who live in an area where there is a lack of facilities or where existing clinics may be understaffed, causing delays in appointment. Doctors may be unable to take smears due either to lack of training or inadequate information on who should have a smear taken and how often. There may also be no laboratory facilities for smear analysis. Some areas have small budgets resulting in restricted policies regarding who should have a smear and sometimes refuse smears to women at risk because the regulation five years have not passed since their last test.

- Women who have had a normal smear some time in the past and think it sufficient. These women may not realize that they

45

should have another one within a prescribed time limit, either because no-one informed them at the time, because they had forgotten, or because they were not recalled.

- Women who are concerned about being examined by a male doctor.
- Women who do not speak English and there is no interpreter available to help them.
- Women with small children who find it difficult to visit a clinic because there is nobody to look after the children.

Problems in obtaining a smear

Nervous women
There may be difficulty in obtaining smears from nervous women because a tight vagina does not easily permit insertion of a speculum and sampling by the spatula. This can be overcome by using smaller speculums, and using differently designed spatulas.

Post-menopausal women
In post-menopausal women, the transformation zone, the area most liable to pre-cancerous change on the cervix, is drawn up high into the cervical canal towards the uterus. This makes it inaccessible to the usual method of sampling when using a standard spatula. This can lead to a falsely negative smear. However, some centres now use a new type of spatula and pipecleaner-like brushes which can reach into the cervical canal and obtain cells. This is an improvement on the previous technique. It also makes it more likely that adenocarcinoma may be detected (see Chapter 10).

Women who have had operations on their cervix
It may be difficult to obtain adequate smears from women who have had operations such as local removal of CIN using diathermy (electrical burning), cryotherapy/cryocautery (freezing), or cone biopsies (cutting a cone of affected tissue from the cervix), because any of these operations may cause narrowing (stenosis) of the endocervical canal and a drawing up of the squamocolumnar junction and transformation zone into the cervical canal. This

means that it is difficult or impossible to scrape cells from this vulnerable site. For the same reason, it may also be difficult to take smears from women whose cervices have been stitched following damage during a difficult delivery. The repair may tighten and distort the cervical surface, thus drawing the transformation zone away from its usual position and making it difficult to sample cells from it.

Pregnant women
It is safe to take smears during pregnancy. However, due to special changes which the cervix undergoes during pregnancy and up to 3 months after childbirth, smears taken at these times may have no endocervical cells, or may show post-natal changes.

Inadequate samples

The problem of not getting enough cells on a slide, poor spreading or staining, or cells being obscured by inflammation or discharge may result in recommendation for a repeat smear. So if your doctor asks you to have another smear shortly after the laboratory results have come back, it does not necessarily mean that there is anything wrong. Most smears are normal and sometimes the cytologists may spot abnormalities which are unconnected with cancer.

These abnormalities may be due to:

- The presence of inflammatory cells caused by a vaginal infection which may not have symptoms such as soreness or foul-smelling discharge.

- The presence of an intrauterine device (IUD or coil) used for contraceptive purposes.

- Obscuring of cervical cells by menstrual discharge if the sample was taken near the time of menstruation.

- Blood-staining if the skin lining was thin, delicate or broke down easily.

- Atrophic cells (hormone [oestrogen] deficient women).

The frequency of smear taking

The frequency with which a woman should have a smear depends upon many factors relevant to each individual case. The first smear should be taken within a year of starting sexual intercourse, no matter what age. Subsequent smears should be taken after an interval not greater than three years. Ideally they should be taken annually.

This recommendation is contradictory to government payment criteria for General Practitioners — who are paid for each smear taken every five years between the ages of 25 and 64 — though such criteria are continually under revision. However, when one considers that there are a number of errors inherent in the cervical smear system (see pages 52-55) and that the subjective impression is of a disease that is becoming more aggressive in its onset, then we consider an annual smear as desirable. however, we recognize that this would place a huge financial burden on the National Health Service, and studies have shown that smears taken every three years strike the best balance in terms of economics and disease prevention.

It is advisable to have a smear within a year of the following circumstances:

● A new sexual partner.

● Discovery of the male partner having other sexual relationships (a cancer-inducing agent may be transmitted from a third party).

● If the previous smear was abnormal or inadequate as indicated by the laboratory (they may even suggest resmearing within six months).

Subsequently, one can revert to smears every three years providing there are no new sexual partners, the relationship is monogamous, and the smear is reported as normal.

Women should have a smear annually or more often as indicated when the following risk factors exist:

- Previous cervical abnormalities such as inflammation, mild or moderate dyskaryosis. If inflammation has been caused by identified infection, this must be treated, cleared and then the smear repeated.

- Previously treated CIN.

- Post-hysterectomy, if the operation was performed as a result of cervical malignancy (CIN or invasive cancer).

- Post-hysterectomy where in rare cases the cervix has not been removed (this is now rare).

- Genital warts on either sexual partner.

- When one's sexual partner has had other partners who have or have had cervical cancer.

- Women of low socioeconomic status.

- Where either partner has a job involving heavy manual labour and frequent handling of toxic chemicals or oil, as these have been linked to increased risk of cervical cancer.

- If one is a heroin abuser.

- If one began sexual intercourse at an early age (under 20).

- If one is taking immunosuppressive drugs (such as azathioprine).

- Presence of signs and symptoms such as pelvic pain or discomfort, discharge, bleeding after sexual intercourse, irregular bleeding, or post-menopausal bleeding at any time.

Women who have had previous treatment for cervical cancer and pre-cancer may remain at risk of this disease recurring for the rest of their lives. Such women have shown their susceptibility to the disease and a second occurrence may be either the result of a new infection due to sexual intercourse or a recurrence of the original disease. These women need to be screened annually by smears. Where any difficulties exist, such as problems with sampling from a narrowed cervical canal, then women should have their smears taken under colposcopic surveillance to increase the rate of detection. The stenosis (narrowing) may have to be treated by cervical dilatation (very occasionally under general anaesthetic) to allow access for smear taking. Ideally, annual colposcopy with simultaneous cytology should be performed on women who have had a hysterectomy for the removal of malignant tissue.

Smears in the post-menopausal woman

Because the cells in post-menopausal women are not easily reached or may not shed or flake off easily, it is advisable to have one repeat smear after a year in case the previous smear failed to detect underlying malignancy. If a post-menopausal woman has ceased having sexual intercourse, she no longer needs a smear after three successive negative results up to her 70th birthday. However, if she resumes intercourse, further smears are necessary at a minimum of three-yearly intervals.

Where old age or other changes make sampling difficult, the situation can be improved by pre-treatment with oestrogen which improves both sampling and quality of smear (see Chapter 10).

Interpreting the smear

Cytology (the study of cells)

Once the cervical cells have been collected, they are sent to a laboratory where they are stained with various dyes and observed under the microscope by an expert in the study of cells—a cytologist. The dyes help to distinguish pre-cancerous cells from normal ones, as the former stain darker and show a different texture from the latter. The degree of change is assessed by looking closely at the particular deviations from normal within the nucleus and cytoplasm, and such changes are the hallmark of potential malignant activity. These observations are used to diagnose the possible presence of the disease or a likelihood of future changes to come.

The terms commonly used to describe the degree of abnormality are **atypia** (mild non-specific change), and **mild, moderate or severe dyskaryosis** (dys = disturbance, karyosis = nucleus). The more dyskaryotic the nucleus of the cell the greater its disturbed growth and malignant potential.

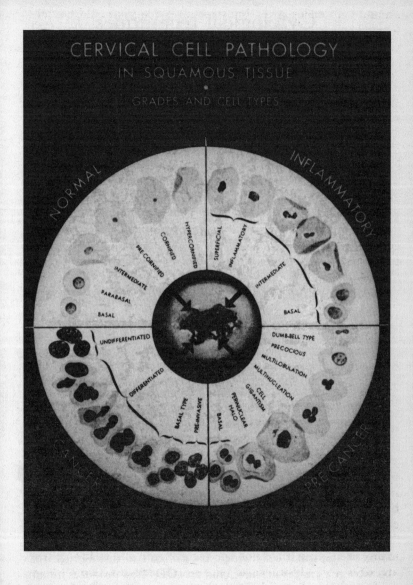

Figure 5 Cytological changes in cervical cells from normal to cancerous.

Cytological techniques

Two kinds of cytological investigations are now available: the static—the examination of stained cells spread on a slide under the microscope, and flow cytometry—examination of cells stained with special dyes and allowed to flow through a glass chamber illuminated with laser light. This light selectively causes cancer cells to fluoresce under the presence of laser light. The automated measurement of the fluorescent light indicates the presence of cancer protein. This technique has only recently been developed and should provide an additional method of detection. Only time will tell if this is to be the screening technique of the future.

There are also new special staining techniques to stain viral and cancer proteins in cells selectively. Such identification is laborious and expensive, and is not generally available as yet. However, until flow cytometry and other automated forms of screening or even a simple blood test for cancer become widely available, the cytologist will continue to be much in demand.

Problems in the cervical smear system

Smear taking — inadequate specimen

The cytologist may experience problems in forming a decision about a smear because an inadequate sample (scanty sample)with no endocervical cells has been collected or the cells may be poorly fixed. This may cause distortion of cell shape, thus making it impossible to analyse the cells correctly.

Unclear smears

The cells may be obscured by discharges containing blood, semen, bacteria or fungi. Infection and inflammation can cause appearance of abnormal cells which are difficult to distinguish from possible pre-cancerous ones, and an IUD often produces inflammatory cells which may also give a false picture. If a woman is having hormonal treatment, such as local oestrogen creams applied in the vagina or is taking oestrogen/progesterone tablets, this may change the appearance of the cells. Similarly, smears taken during and up to six to eight weeks after pregnancy, may present a different appearance as may smears after recent operative treatments on the cervix. Doctors should mention any of these when they send samples to the cytologist. Oestrogen deficiency, which may occur with advancing years, is reflected in changes in the cells which become *atrophic*. Severe atrophic changes in post-menopausal women may mimic cancer and have to be distinguished from cancer.

Human error in reading the smears

On the whole very few errors in reading smears are made. However, errors can and do occur giving false negative results. Of course, if a cytologist has to screen cells for many hours with a likely detection rate of between 2 and 5 positive results per thousand, it is understandable that their detection rate is not going to be 100 per cent, particularly if the abnormality is slight. Since such reporting depends on human judgement, the presence or absence of abnormalities and their subsequent reporting can differ between cytologists. Occasionally, a cell may look malignant but on closer inspection this may be due to other causes. This is a false positive error. Overall, smear misreporting is thought to occur in between 2 and 14 per cent of cases, depending on laboratory staff experience, availability, and workload.

Administrative errors

These can include a mix-up of slides, poor writing, wrong labelling or, after processing, reading the wrong smear from the tray. Sometimes, screeners report without proper name or identification number; there may be an error in transcription by the typist; a wrong address put on the envelope, or the letter may even get lost in the post.

It is important that an efficient administrative procedure is set in motion to obtain accurate analysis rapidly and to ensure that women waiting for their results are informed as soon as possible. To understand how things might go wrong, it is worth looking briefly at a typical administrative system.

To start with, the slides of the cervical smears need to be labelled with a patient's name, date of birth, the date of sampling, and the date of collection. Accompanying multi-copy forms need to be filled out, and various data concerning menstruation, pregnancy, previous smears, operations, and hormonal treatments may be needed because they can and do affect the appearance of cells and their interpretation by the cytologist.

When the cytologist has analysed the smear, a copy of his/her report has to be sent to the person who has carried out that test (i.e. the doctor or nurse) and a copy is also retained by the laboratory. The remaining copy is sent to the local health authority.

Notification of smear results

In an ideal world all women would be informed of the result of their smear test quickly and accurately, and given a recommendation concerning further testing and treatment. However, the pressure on the system is such that it can be as much as eight or ten weeks later before the woman hears her result, and, in some health authorities, women are only informed if their smear is positive (abnormal). The problem with this is that it doesn't take into account that the woman may move without leaving a forwarding address, the doctor or nurse taking the smear may write her address down incorrectly, or the letter may get lost in the post.

However, there are ways in which a woman can help the system so that she gets her result. She must make sure she informs her GP or clinic if she changes her address; she can make sure that the person taking her smear gets her address and other details correct and she should 'phone her GP or clinic to find out her results for herself.

Accuracy in the detection of pre-cancer by cervical smears

We have described many possible difficulties that may arise in reporting the results of cervical smears. The errors which occur can be divided into false positive smears (those reporting an abnormality which on rechecking does not exist) and the more common false negative smears (failure to detect existing abnormality) or a failure to report at all. Despite the inherent problems with the system, most smears are correctly reported. There are occasional major hiccups, such as the well-publicized incident which occured in Liverpool in September 1987 where more than 900 smears over a four year period were incorrectly reported as negative. Depending on the centres taking the smears and the laboratories reporting them, the accuracy of results is between 70 and 98 per cent.

The smear result

Abnormal smears

A smear may be reported as abnormal if it exhibits any change which differs from normal. Inflammatory changes and non-cancerous cell abnormalities occur frequently in response to a variety of bacterial, viral and fungal infections. Where possible, these should be identified and treated and the smear repeated until a normal result is obtained. If the abnormality persists despite the treatment or if no treatable cause of the abnormality is found, the cervix and vulvo-vaginal area should be examined with a colposcope (binocular microscope) to try and identify further the reason and source of the abnormality. (See chapter 4.)

Positive smears

The reporting of a positive smear means that identifiable pre-cancerous or cancerous cells (a pre-cancerous finding is far more likely) are reported by the cytologist. This does not always mean that cancer exists. However, in this situation the cervix must be inspected using a colposcope. This is because while the smear can give a picture of what is happening in the cells obtained from the cervix, it cannot provide the information of such details as the position, spread and depth of the pre-cancer or cancer on the cervix. Such information is vital in order to be able to correctly determine the nature of the disease and to recommend suitable treatment. Using current accepted terminology a positive smear is one which has severely dyskaryotic cells. In order to find out more about abnormalities on your cervix, your GP or clinic may recommend a number of further tests which are described in the next chapter.

Terms used to describe cytological findings

Different centres evolved various terminologies for their findings and, similarly, different countries have adopted their own set of descriptions of cervical cells. Cytologists, pathologists and clinicians were often confused by the terminologies used by their colleagues in the same countries and even more so by colleagues in different countries. It was, therefore, essential to introduce a common nomenclature which would be understood by all concerned, not least of all the patient and her GP. In order to attempt to standardize the terminology, the British Society for Clinical Cytology (BSCC) has recently defined and recommended a set of terms for general use in interpreting cervical smears. It is difficult or well nigh impossible for some of the patients to understand the terms used, the reason and need for re-smearing and what exactly is happening to them or what is wrong with them.

At present, when the smears have been analysed by cytologists working in the British National Health Service, their findings are reported in four sections on a smear report (see sections 21 to 24 on the smear report in the appendix on p.198). In the *cytology report*, the cytologist uses various terms to describe cellular changes indicating or describing the presence of foreign organisms including viruses, bacteria, and fungi (See the following pages, 57-62, for examples of cytological terms and follow-up recommendations).

Some centres prefer to report smear results in terms of *class*. These correspond to the following terms in cytology and histology:

- Class 1 and 2 smears correspond to normal or inflammatory changes, and also squamous metaplasia.

- Class 3 smear corresponds to mild dyskaryosis (Mild dysplasia CIN 1).
- Class 4 smear corresponds to moderate dyskaryosis (Moderate dysplasia CIN 2).
- Class 5 smear corresponds to severe dyskaryosis (Severe dysplasia CIN 3).

Cytology terms

- Actinomycetes — these fungi, when they are present, are usually found in the presence of intrauterine devices (IUDs). If they cause inflammatory changes, the IUD should be removed and treatment with antibiotics may be necessary to clear the infection. At present, actinomycetes have not been implicated in cervical cancer and normal recall is recommended.

- Air-dried smear — Cells are poorly fixed and therefore interpretation impossible and a repeat smear is necessary.

- Anucleate squames — Large flat cells without a nucleus sometimes found when the cervix is prolapsed. Currently normal recall recommended, however some observers have hinted that these cells may be a hallmark of forthcoming pre-cancer and should be re-examined with further smears and colposcopy within a year.

- Atrophic smear — Thin, shrivelled cells reflecting deficiency of oestrogen common in post-menopausal women but also present in other conditions, e.g. when the ovaries are removed (oophorectomy), or where there is a low oestrogen output. Hormonal replacement treatment may be recommended. Normal recall recommended.

- Atypia or atypical cells — Cellular changes which are very mild. A repeat smear is recommended in six months. If it persists, colposcopy is recommended.

- Atypical squamous metaplasia — This indicates that normal skin cells around the entry of the cervical canal (endocervical cells) have been replaced by an atypical squamous epithelium.

This is often the result of inflammation. There is a need to repeat the smear at a future date as suggested by the laboratory to exclude any further abnormality.

- Candida — See thrush.

- Carcinoma *in situ* — Profound and advanced cell disturbance indicating there exists at the very least a carcinoma *in situ* where there are such advanced changes in the cell that they rarely revert to normal and progression to invasive cancer is likely in one in three cases unless treatment is provided. The cytologist (who only sees cells and not tissues) cannot be sure whether or not the carcinoma has invaded deeper into the tissues and is now an invasive cancer rather than one which is *in situ*. All that can be reported on seeing such cells is that malignancy exists and is capable of, or may already have, spread to deeper and to other parts of the body. Colposcopy and biopsy (see below) are urgently needed to identify and confirm or deny the suspicion of invasion and to determine the spread and depth of cellular change. Appropriate treatment is recommended as a result of this combined investigation. Invasion is defined as being when the carcinoma cells break through the deeper layer of the cervical skin (basement membrane) and invade the underlying tissues and lymphatic and blood vessels.

- Cervical biopsy — A sample of tissue taken from the cervix using biopsy forceps, preferably under colposcopic vision. A biopsy is recommended when cells are reported as highly suspicious. As the cervix has very few nerve fibres sampling is virtually painless and no anaesthetic is needed.

- Clue cells — Non-malignant change in the cells due to an infection by Gardnerella (bacterium which sometimes lives in the vagina).

- Colposcopy (colpo = vagina, scopy = look) — Inspection of the cervix with a colposcope (a high-powered binocular microscope) to identify the position, size and extent of an area of abnormality whose presence is suspected from the smear result. Such inspection is indicated when abnormal cells are reported by the cytologist or if the case history suggests a likelihood of cancer despite the presence of a normal smear. Inspection of the cervix and use of special dyes (normal saline followed by acetic acid and occasionally iodine) helps to visualize abnormal areas on the cervix and enables accurately targeted tiny samples (biopsies) to be removed for histology (see histology).

- Dyskaryosis (dys = bad, karyosis = nucleus) — Alteration within the normal arrangement of the cell nucleus. It can be mild, moderate or severe and may become a potential prelude to cancer. Mild, moderate, and severe dyskaryosis usually corresponds to the histological terms CIN 1, CIN 2 and CIN 3 respectively. The possibility of progression to malignancy increases with the degree of dyskaryosis.

- Dysplasia (dys = bad, plasia = formation) — This term was initially used by cytologists to describe cell disturbances and had a similar meaning to dyskaryosis. It is now used to describe tissue abnormalities and has been displaced by dyskaryosis as a term to describe disturbances in the cell nucleus.

- Endocervical cells — Cells from the cervical canal. Their presence indicates that the cervical canal has been sampled. Their absence on a smear may possibly indicate inadequate sampling.

- Endometrial cells (the endometrium is the lining of the uterus) — Cells from the uterus which are shed during menstruation. Their presence in the smear at other times, especially in the second half of the cycle or in post-menopausal women, indicates a need for further investigation such as colposcopy and possibly a need for dilatation and curettage (scraping the endometrium) of the uterus to exclude endometrial carcinoma. Occasionally endometrial cells may appear on a smear following pregnancy or if an intrauterine device (IUD) has been inserted.

- Glandular endocervical cells — Identified by staining for the presence of mucin. Rarely reported but may indicate an adenocarcinoma of the cervix — this very rare form of cancer appears to be on the increase and it may be advisable for laboratories to start routine staining for mucin.

- Glandular neoplasia (neoplasia = cancer, neo = new, plasia = formation) — Chunks of cells from glandular endometrial epithelium with malignant appearance. Curettage and colposcopy recommended.

- Herpes virus — The presence of such a virus is indicated by a report of multinucleated giant cells. Its presence can be confirmed by using special techniques and a further follow-up with cytology is recommended to exclude presence of pre-cancer/cancer. It was thought at one time that this virus causes cervical cancer but studies have not substantiated this.

- Histology — Examination of biopsy (tissue samples) to identify the presence of abnormal cells, their degree of abnormality, distribution and depth of penetration into the tissues, blood vessels and lymphatics.

- HPV — Human Papilloma Virus, commonly abbreviated to wart virus (See the wart virus).

- Inadequate specimen — Refers to a lack of cells or poorly fixed cells on the slide and a repeat smear is necessary.

- Inflammation/inflammatory changes — Changes in cervical cells which in addition may be obscured on the slide by white blood cells produced in response to infection; there may also be cellular changes caused by the presence of infective agents such as bacteria, viruses, or fungi. Such infections are occasionally identified on the smear, or if suspected by presence of inflammatory cells they should be identified by further bacteriological and virological investigation and treated. It is important to repeat smears within six months and if inflammation persists the cervix must be examined with a colposcope to exclude underlying CIN.

- Koilocytes — Cells whose nucleus appear to be surrounded by a halo of cytoplasm. This change has been shown to be a result of infection or some injury to the cell, for instance caused by a wart virus. Such cells may be associated with pre-cancerous/cancerous changes.

- Malignant crowded columnar epithelium — Cells from the endocervix are highly suspicious and suggest adenocarcinoma of the cervix.

- Metaplasia (meta = half, plasia = formation) — See Squamous metaplasia).

- Microinvasive carcinoma — A cancer which has penetrated beneath the skin of the cervix and is invading deeper tissues.

- Mild, moderate dyskaryosis — See Dyskaryosis.

- Monilia — See Thrush.

- Severe dyskaryosis — See Dyskaryosis.

- Squamous metaplasia — Describes the transitional changes which occur during the replacement of endocervical epithelium with squamous epithelium on the surface of the cervix. This is a natural process which begins at puberty and may continue until a woman is in her 40s. See also Atypical squamous metaplasia.

- Thrush (reported on smear results as **candida,** a fungus infection, or **monilia**) — A fungal infection frequently occurring in the vagina and cervix which may cause a thick white discharge and intense itching, but can be present without causing any such symptoms. It may give rise to inflammatory cells on smears which may hide existing and non-exfoliating precancerous cells on the cervix, so treatment must be followed with a repeat smear to ensure a more reliable cytological report.

  Candida can also exist invisibly (or occasionally white spots) on the penis and foreskin when it occasionally causes itching and soreness, and can be transferred during sexual intercourse.

- Trichomonas vaginalis — A sexually transmitted infection whose presence may be detected on the smear by its heart shape structure and long tail. It is an anaerobic infection (it likes warm, moist, dark and airless places) and the vagina is an ideal place for it to live. It may exist without any signs or symptoms, often for many years, but it may cause green offensive discharge and produce soreness. Smears taken in the presence of such an infection may contain inflammatory cells and in such conditions it is necessary to treat and repeat the smear between three and six months after treatment.

- Uterine curettage (also known as D & C — dilatation and curettage) — Scraping the lining of the uterus with a curette (a long thin metal spoon) for histological and cytological examination. This is indicated when cancerous changes are suspected in the uterine lining suggested by endometrial cells appearing in the smear.

- Viral changes — This refers to changes in the cells produced by viruses, e.g., herpes virus or human papilloma wart virus. Such cells are known as koilocytes (See also Koilocytes).

- Wart virus infection — This refers to the human papilloma virus (HPV) whose presence is shown by koilocytic cells and can be accompanied by mild, moderate or severe dyskaryosis. Such smears should be followed up by colposcopy (which is described fully in chapter 4).

Chapter 4

Colposcopy, punch biopsy, cone biopsy and loop excision

- A colposcope is an illuminated binocular microscope. It is used to give a magnified view of the cervix when a smear or case history suggests the presence of an abnormality.

- Colposcopy is a painless and safe procedure performed in under half an hour. No anaesthetic is required.

- Small tissue samples (biopsies) are taken from areas of suspected abnormality to discover the depth and nature of the abnormality.

- Cellular abnormalities observed by the histologists are graded in terms of cervical intraepithelial neoplasia (CIN), as CIN 1 (mild), CIN 2 (moderate), and CIN 3 (severe abnormality).

- CIN conditions are pre-cancerous, i.e. they have the potential to progress on to cancer. The more severe the CIN, the more likely it will become cancerous.

- Carcinoma *in situ* is a condition where the pre-cancerous cells have become cancerous but are confined to the cervical skin.

- In microinvasive carcinoma, the malignant cells have spread beyond the cervical skin membrane.

- Invasive cancer describes an invasion of greater than three millimetres beyond the basement membrane, possibly involving blood vessels and lymphatic channels.

● Combining cytology (smears) with colposcopy and histology increases the chances of detecting abnormalities from 70 to 98 per cent.

The tests most frequently used in detecting the nature and extent of abnormalities on the cervix are colposcopy, biopsy (sometimes called punch biopsy) and cone biopsy. We shall look at colposcopy first, as this is the test you will probably undergo first.

Colposcopy

The History of Colposcopy

Colposcopy has only recently become available as a diagnostic investigation in Britain. In the 1950s and 60s, cone biopsy (sometimes called conization) of the cervix (removal of a cone-shaped piece of tissue from the cervix) was the routine diagnostic procedure for all women with severely abnormal smears. This was because other diagnostic techniques such as random cervical biopsies were insufficiently precise and colposcopy was not available.

The colposcope was invented as long ago as 1925 in Germany by an innovative gynaecologist called Hans Hinselmann. He took an ordinary microscope, mounted it on a movable arm, endowed it with binocular vision, gave it brilliant illumination, and, with a speculum gently inserted into the vagina so as to open it, he was able to inspect the cervix. He thought that the beginnings of cervical cancer might occur as small ulcers, or tumours, which could be detected using suitable magnification. He used the colposcope for the inspection of vaginal, vulvovaginal and cervical areas and was then able to see and describe the appearance of various cervices. He saw the malignant lesions (abnormal, diseased area) and demonstrated the effect of various dyes, such as acetic acid, which brought out the abnormal areas as white patches, and Lugol's iodine, which, when applied to the cervix, stained all the normal cervical skin and vaginal epithelium deeply brown. (This is known as Schiller's test.)

For many years colposcopy was mostly confined to Germany and not widely used in other countries as a useful diagnostic tool, partly because little was known about it, and also because of the difficulty and cost of equipment and training. Furthermore, the detection of cervical abnormalities by cytology, which developed in parallel with colposcopy, was simpler and cheaper than colposcopy. It was not until much later that doctors appreciated that a combination of the two techniques was essential to improve the detection, correct diagnosis, and treatment of the disease.

For some 25 years colposcopy was mostly confined to German-speaking countries. However, after the Second World War, Hinselmann went to South America where his colposcopic techniques became popular.

In Britain, British gynaecologists became interested in colposcopy in the 1960s and the British Colposcopy Group which has now become the British Society for Colposcopy and Cervical Pathology (BSCCP) was formed in 1971. The BSCCP has over 700 members and is still growing. The main reason for the increase in popularity was that pre-cancers were occuring in younger women and a need arose for accurate definition of the abnormal area and subsequent optimal local treatment so hysterectomy could be avoided where possible, thereby preserving a woman's reproductive functions and avoiding unnecessary major surgery.

The colposcopic examination

If a smear has been reported as abnormal and the cytologist has suggested colposcopy, the examination will usually be performed in hospital by gynaecological consultants or registrars. It is preferable to avoid having colposcopy when menstruating as this may interfere with the doctor being able to see the cervix. Also, the vaginal area is more sensitive during menstruation and there may be discomfort during examination. However, if necessary, colposcopy can be carried out during menstruation. It can be carried out in the presence of an intrauterine device (IUD).

Colposcopy can also be performed during pregnancy and will not cause any harm to the mother or baby.

On arrival at a colposcopy clinic, there is often a time delay in waiting for colposcopy because of the pressure on the clinics. Appointments vary in length according to each individual's case history and the need for explanation and discussion may be time consuming.

A thorough history should be taken which should include questions on general health, contraceptive methods, hormone treatment, gynaecological health, post-menopausal bleeding, details of periods including the date of the last one, past or present existence of genital warts on oneself and current and previous partners, details of pregnancies and sexual history, occupation (your own and partner's), details of previous smears and any subsequent treatments, smoking habits, and whether there is a family history of cancer, cervical or otherwise. Such information will provide vital clues to a likely presence of an abnormality and can increase the alertness of the colposcopist when searching for what may be tiny and yet highly suspect areas of abnormality.

The patient is examined in a similar position as for a smear and the whole process takes around fifteen minutes and is usually painless. In some centres the patients' legs may be placed high up on stirrups during the examination.

In large hospitals and teaching clinics you may be asked if student doctors and nurses other than the colposcopist can be present during the examination as part of their training. It is helpful if there is a nurse present to reassure and look after the patient. You can of course refuse to have anyone present other than the person taking the sample.

The examination should include the vulva, vagina, cervix, and the cervical canal, as far as it can be seen. The vulvovaginal area is first inspected for the possible presence of any abnormalities and in particular for the presence of any genital warts which may signify a possible existence of pre-malignant disease on the cervix. A closed speculum is gently passed into the vagina, then opened gently and the inside walls of the vagina inspected. When the cervix is revealed the speculum is held in position. At this time, cervical smears and high vaginal swabs may be taken. After the samples are obtained, a saline (salt) solution is applied to the cervix. This brings out and improves the inspection of blood vessels on the cervix. The variation in the presence, appearance and distribution of blood vessels gives information on the possible presence of disease. After this, the cervix is painted with a

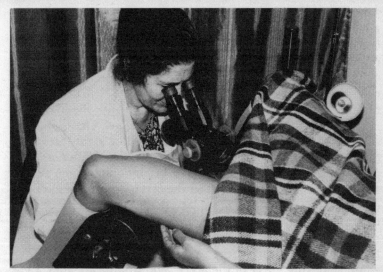

Fig 6(a)

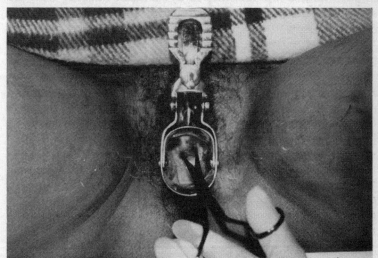

Fig 6(b)

Figure 6 a) A colposcopic examination. b) Colposcopic examination of the cervical canal, which is opened by forceps.

3 or 5 per cent **acetic acid** solution. This may cause a brief and mild stinging sensation. The acetic acid makes the previously invisible abnormalities begin to appear slowly as areas of varying degrees of whiteness, textures, and patterns.

The cervical canal is gently opened using a special pair of delicate forceps and more acetic acid is added to help see how far the abnormality has ascended into the canal and whether or not it is possible to see how far and where it stops. Occasionally a solution of iodine may also be applied. Iodine stains brown all the areas which contain sugar and most normal squamous skin cells covering the vagina and cervix do contain glycogen and do stain brown. Abnormal areas on the cervix, normal endocervical epithelium, immature metaplasia (early stages of change from columnar to squamous epithelium) and occasionally also normal but very old and ageing areas, do not contain any glycogen and do not stain, and appear as pale yellow or white areas. The white colouring effect of the acetic acid disappears after a few minutes unless it is maintained by constant dabbing with the solution. Both acetic acid and iodine are, therefore, useful diagnostic dyes.

Colposcopy for all

At present, colposcopy is performed almost exclusively by hospital doctors and is too expensive for the majority of GPs to perform, yet they are in an ideal position to carry out this form of screening. It is something of a Catch 22 situation with the colposcopic kit being expensive because the market is so small yet if every GP bought one they would be very cheap. Currently, hospitals are doing virtually all colposcopy examinations but lack the number of staff to cater for the needs of the community, hence the long waiting lists for evaluation of abnormal smears. Another problem is one of training as in the hands of an inexperienced colposcopist, colposcopy can be useless and even dangerously misleading. Experience is vital to recognize many of the very subtle changes observed under the colposcope. For example, it can be very difficult to recognize a microinvasive carcinoma where the cancerous cells invade quickly and are covered by a thin layer of normal cells which may obscure them. However, an expert eye can detect them. As there are so few colposcopy centres, it is difficult for doctors to gain experience, particularly if they do not work in an area where there is a colposcopy service and where there is a consultant willing to teach.

The demand for colposcopy is rising for several reasons— more women are found to have abnormal smears which require colposcopic evaluation, more women are having treatment which requires colposcopic follow-up, and some women with normal smears but suspicious case histories also need to be examined to discover a hidden disease. If the cervix looks suspicious to the doctor's naked eye, colposcopy may be recommended with or without a preceding smear test. Abnormalities on the vulva and vagina are also looked for, especially for the presence of genital warts which are sometimes too small to be seen with the naked eye. However, biopsies from these highly sensitive areas are not easy to obtain without discomfort to the patient so they are sampled either under a local anaesthetic injected into the skin or when the patient is under general anaesthetic. At the time of examination, diagrams are drawn and notes are made for reference of all the suspect areas and position of biopsies.

Punch biopsy

Punch biopsies are very small amounts of tissue taken from abnormal areas and sent for histological examination. These are used to identify the presence, distribution and depth of the abnormality observed by colposcopy. As the cervix has very few sensory nerve fibres, taking or 'punching out' small samples from its surface is virtually painless (samples taken are approximately the size of a grain of a rice!). Using the colposcope as a visual guide, samples are taken with special biopsy forceps. The biopsies are targeted on the abnormal area, which is frequently on the transformation zone but, on rare occasions, the biopsy may miss the abnormality, or the sample may be too small or crushed to permit adequate reporting (thus requiring a repeat biopsy). The biopsy should go through and beyond the skin into the underlying cervical tissue in order to confirm the presence of abnormal cells throughout the thickness of the skin. The biopsies are fixed in special preserving solution and sent together with supporting documentation and smear results for histological examination.

Bleeding from the biopsy area can be stopped with silver nitrate sticks. This takes a few minutes and occasionally produces a mild period-like cramp which soon passes. It is advisable to avoid intercourse for the next week to allow the area to heal, and to avoid using any internal vaginal tampons as they may rub against the biopsied area, delay healing, and increase bleeding and the chance of infection. Swimming and baths should be avoided for a week following the biopsy.

On the rare occasions when bleeding occurs one or two weeks following the biopsy, it is advisable to go to one's GP or the person who took the biopsy. The bleeding can be stopped by application of the silver nitrate sticks.

Cone biopsy

There are several circumstances in which colposcopy must be followed by further investigation such as cone biopsy. One such situation is when adenocarcinoma of the cervix (cancer which occurs in the folds of the columnar epithelium) is suspected. Such suspicion is aroused when the cytologist observes and reports 'malignant columnar cells' on the smear. Cone biopsy is required because there are no colposcopic criteria yet defined for describing such abnormalities. Cone biopsy is the only way of knowing for sure whether adenocarcinoma exists and whether it is confined locally or has spread out beyond the margins of the cone into the deeper tissues.

Other more common situations which necessitate the use of cone biopsy include:

● When there is a positive cervical smear result but there is no abnormality seen on colposcopy.

- When colposcopy cannot reveal the area of abnormality in its entirety, for example, when it disappears into the endocervical canal and the top of it cannot be seen.

- When the biopsy has shown the presence of a possible microinvasive or invasive carcinoma.

- When there are no colposcopic facilities.

In all of these circumstances a cone biopsy is essential.

A cone biopsy involves the removal of a cone-shaped piece of tissue from the cervix to determine the source and depth of abnormality and, in some cases, to remove the entire diseased area (i.e. diagnosis and cure may be simultaneous). However, it may also show that the cells reach beyond the limits of excision and are likely to have been left behind in the cervix and may require a deeper and more radical treatment—a repeated bigger cone biopsy, or even hysterectomy.

The removal of the tissue usually involves hospital admission and a general anaesthetic. In women over 40, there may also be simultaneous D and C (D = dilatation C = curettage—i.e.

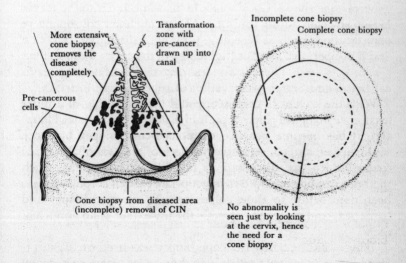

More extensive cone biopsy removes the disease completely

Transformation zone with pre-cancer drawn up into canal

Pre-cancerous cells

Cone biopsy from diseased area (incomplete) removal of CIN

Incomplete cone biopsy
Complete cone biopsy

No abnormality is seen just by looking at the cervix, hence the need for a cone biopsy

Figure 7 Complete and incomplete cone biopsies.

71

opening the cervix and scraping the cervical canal and uterus). In this way, most of the tissues likely to be involved in a potential malignancy can be removed and analysed by the histologist. The area to be cut out is identified by colposcopic visualization (or by naked eye) and staining of the cervix with iodine to show up the abnormal areas indicated in the colposcopy report. The process of cutting out the tissues causes a variable amount of bleeding. The remaining tissues require stitching in order to stop the flow of blood.

The whole procedure requires a hospital stay of around three days. After the operation, there is some pain, bleeding and discomfort, and sexual intercourse should be avoided until after the follow-up visit six weeks later.

Some hospitals are able to perform cone biopsies using a sophisticated laser which works like a knife. Here, the laser cuts out the cone and coagulates the tissues on the surface of the area from which the cone has been removed at the same time, thus preventing bleeding. This technique is a great improvement on the standard cold knife procedure as it can be performed in less than half an hour, often without the need for hospitalization, or general anaesthesia. Local anaesthetic is injected into the cervix to stop any pain during conization. There are fewer post-operative complications such as bleeding, prolonged discharge, infection and post-operative stenosis (tightening of the cervical canal) than if a knife is used. There is also less destruction of normal cervical tissue and better preservation of reproductive function.

With the advent of colposcopy and the possibility of a more accurate cytological colposcopic and histological analysis of biopsies, it has become possible to replace cone biopsy by more sophisticated and conservative methods of removal of abnormal tissue (which are discussed in the following chapter). Such methods can be employed in appropriate cases if colposcopy has been used before to allow colposcopically directed biopsy and to identify and diagnose correctly the full extent of an abnormal area.

Where until recently the cone biopsy was used on all suspicious smears it is now used only in those cases where colposcopy is unsatisfactory. This includes cases where the full extent of the abnormal cervical skin or epithelium cannot be seen or where an abnormal smear result is not accompanied by a relevant colposcopic impression. Cone biopsy is also necessary where a punch biopsy (see later) fails to explain a positive smear or if a microinvasive or frankly invasive cancer is suspected.

Problems of cone biopsy

Other than bleeding, there should generally be few problems following a cone biopsy. However, risk of infection is raised following all surgery. Occasionally, narrowing of the cervical canal after healing makes it difficult for menstrual discharge to be released, and this causes period pains when there is no discharge. Another problem associated with stenosis after surgery is that it can become difficult to collect endocervical cells during follow-up smears. Special instruments may be needed to sample such cells or, in extreme cases, re-admission to hospital to have the cervical canal dilated may be necessary.

Pregnancy and fertility (see also chapter 10)

A cone biopsy may damage the cervix and can lead to difficulty in maintaining a pregnancy (cervical incompetence), resulting in miscarriage. This can be overcome by stitching up the cervix in early pregnancy and removing the shirodkar stitch just before delivery. Sometimes during delivery, the conized cervix fails to dilate fully and a Caesarean section will be necessary. There is a spontaneous abortion rate of between 12 and 22 per cent as a result of cone biopsy at an earlier date. Premature labour also occurs in between 7.5 and 9.5 per cent of women who have had cone biopsy, and low birth weight infants are born in 21 per cent of cases. However, it should be emphasized that the vast majority of pregnancies in women who have had cone biopsies progress quite normally.

Before the advent of colposcopy, cone biopsy was the standard technique for investigation of cervical cancer. However, with more information gained by colposcopy, cone biopsy does not need to be performed as often as before and the technique is only used for the few cases mentioned before. In the past, cone biopsy involved the removal of a much larger area than nowadays to ensure that the whole of the diseased area was removed. This may have affected the capacity of the cervical canal and its mucus to facilitate the transport of sperm subsequently and thus fertility may have been impaired. However, when a colposcopically guided cone biopsy allows for a minimal and yet complete removal of all abnormal tissue with minimal damage to the cervix, the likelihood of fertility being affected is small. However, in the event of this happening, it may be necessary to dilate the cervical canal to facilitate sperm passage. If this fails, artificial insemination or *in vitro* fertilization (the so-called 'test-tube baby' method) techniques may be necessary.

In conclusion, although many women will need a cone biopsy to investigate/treat a cervical abnormality, we would stress that it should not be feared as such biopsies can nowadays be accurately targeted under colposcopic surveillance resulting in minimal damage and discomfort. Laser conization, where available, further reduces the likelihood of problems.

Loop excision

A technique known as diathermy loop excision (DLE) or Large Loop Excision of the Transformation Zone (LLETZ) has grown in popularity in the last year or so. It may eventually replace punch and cone (knife and laser) biopsies, as a way of taking samples for histological examination. It may also replace some of the local ablative removal techniques mentioned in chapter 5.

The technique involves using an electrically-heated wire loop to remove a section of tissue from the surface of the cervix, thereby taking a larger sample of tissue than a punch biopsy while being not as destructive and damaging as a cone biopsy.

What the biopsy reveals (Histological analysis)

Examination of the sample obtained by punch biopsy, cone biopsy or loop excision is known as histology, and is carried out by an expert known as a histologist (sometimes referred to as a histo-pathologist).

The biopsies are fixed and stained with various diagnostic dyes and slices of such tissues are examined under the microscope. Whereas cytology alone allows for description of the disturbance confined within the cells, histology allows for an extended description of the disturbance both within the cell and their distribution, location, spread and penetration of affected cells into the tissues, sometimes revealing penetration into the blood vessels and lymphatic channels, depending on the depth of the biopsy.

Cervical intraepithelial neoplasia (CIN)

If the histologist sees any abnormalities, they are described in terms of **cervical intraepithelial neoplasia (CIN),** which literally means 'new growth within the skin of the cervix'. Used in this way, CIN describes the degree of the cervical abnormality when it is still in a pre-cancerous condition. CIN covers the complete range of epithelial (skin) abnormalities of the cervix from the mildest form to carcinoma *in situ* which is when the cells have become cancerous but have not spread beyond the cervical skin. To make the diagnosis of CIN more meaningful it is followed by a number which indicates the degree of abnormality. Approximately 60-70 per cent of CIN 1 cases revert to normal. CIN 1 refers to cells which are abnormal in that they have minor changes in cell structure which are the first signs of pre-cancer. CIN 1 usually corresponds with the cytological observation of mild dyskaryosis found on the cervical smear and is sometimes referred to as mild **dysplasia** (the term commonly used until recently in cytology but now reserved for histology). However, occasionally the smear may identify mild dyskaryosis while the biopsy shows CIN 2 or CIN 3 (more advanced types of pre-cancer) and vice versa.

The next stage in severity is CIN 2, which usually correlates with moderate dyskaryosis (although, as with CIN 1, there are occasional exceptions), where there are more advanced changes than in CIN 1, although they may regress. In such cases, the laboratory may advise a repeat smear or colposcopy.

In CIN 3 (severe dyskaryosis or carcinoma *in situ*), there are definite changes of pre-malignancy, and one in three cases will progress to invasive cancer unless the abnormal cells are removed. In this situation the laboratory will recommend urgent colposcopy and biopsy to determine the extent of the abnormality and whether there is any invasion. It is unlikely for CIN to give rise to any signs or symptoms, so the only way of detecting them is by regular screening of the asymptomatic population.

The reason that cytological (smears) and histological (biopsy results, i.e. CIN) may be at variance with each other is because it is possible for all the CIN stages to exist on one cervix.

On rare occasions moderate dyskaryosis (CIN 2) can develop directly into invasive cancer. Several studies have shown that around 30 to 35 per cent of pre-cancers regress spontaneously. The milder forms have the highest regression rates. However, all forms of abnormalities need to be followed up to ensure either their disappearance or, if the abnormality persists, to remove it.

Carcinoma *in situ* CIS

The cytological and histological finding of the most severe degree of pre-cancerous change in cells and tissues still confined to the cervical skin is often called **carcinoma *in situ*** and is equivalent to CIN 3. At this point the pre-cancerous cells are now cancerous, malignant, and, in up to one in three cases, the cells will invade sooner or later. The progression to invasion may take a few months or several years and it is impossible to predict the time span of any individual case if the CIN 3 is left untreated. Carcinoma *in situ* is the point of no return—if it gets any further, local treatments may not be possible. At this stage, the cervical cells appear to be quite different from normal cells, and show abnormal division on biopsy.

Microinvasive carcinoma

Biopsies can also reveal the presence of a microinvasion and urgent treatment should be recommended. In microinvasion, the cells, which have by now acquired a high malignancy potential, have broken through the basement membrane (the tissue barrier separating the skin from the underlying deeper tissue containing blood vessels and lymphatic channels). These cells are called the microinvasive cells. Once beneath the basement membrane, they continue to multiply and spread deeper under the skin. As long as their presence does not reach deeper than three millimetres from the basement of the membrane at the point of invasion, and they have not yet entered any of the lymphatic or blood vessels, these cells fall in the category of microinvasion. A cone biopsy will now be needed to determine (and often to simultaneously remove) the extent of the abnormality.

Invasive carcinoma

Where this situation is suspected, a cone biopsy is needed in order to determine whether or not malignant cells have reached deeper than three millimetres from the basement membrane, and if the lymphatic and blood channels have been involved. This is because once they break into the blood and lymph systems, the invasive carcinoma can be spread to the rest of the body by a process called **metastasis**. (Invasive carcinoma is described in more detail later on.)

Progression from pre-cancer to malignancy

Unfortunately, it is not yet possible to determine which individual cases of milder CIN abnormalities are likely to regress or which will progress to become invasive cancer. Neither is it possible to predict how long it will take to reach the latter stage. Therefore, all abnormalities should be regarded as having a potential for malignancy and should be investigated fully by smear, colposcopy and biopsy. If a mild abnormality is found but seems not to warrant treatment, it needs to be followed up by repeated investigation as above.

Notification of colposcopy and cone biopsy results

After colposcopy, and often before the result of a biopsy, other than cone biopsy, is known, the colposcopist may be in a position to tell the patient whether she is likely to have a pre-cancer or cancer present and what form of treatment (if any) is likely to be suitable, subject to the findings of biopsy. In circumstances where colposcopy is unsatisfactory, this information has to await further investigations, for instance, cone biopsy.

All the information from a colposcopic examination is subject to biopsy results and can only be provisional. Surprises have been known to happen. For instance, a small area which looks to the colposcopist like a mild abnormality, may on histological examination of the biopsy show the disease to be more advanced both in severity of nuclear change and in the depth of its penetration, or both. In contrast, a severely dyskaryotic smear may be shown on colposcopy and biopsy to have come from an extremely localized and minute area, or in fact not be visible at all. A repeat colposcopy, and possibly even conization, may be necessary to identify the source of the abnormal cells. This is why most colposcopists are rather guarded in giving definite information until the biopsy results are known because in order to be accurate, they need the information from the combined investigations.

The histologist's report on the biopsy or cone biopsy is sent to the colposcopist who took the sample. These results are then viewed in conjunction with the patient's case history and the decision made regarding treatment, usually by the colposcopist, or by a consultant gynaecologist. The patient should be informed of the result, whether treatment is required, and what form it will take. The time taken for the results to come through depends on each area. It may take only a couple of days, as long as a couple of weeks or even longer than that.

Cervicography

The most recent innovation in visualization of the cervix, is **cervicography**. This technique allows for photographs of the cervix to be taken using a specialized camera. As for colposcopy, a speculum is inserted, the cervix is painted with acetic acid and appropriate time allowed for any abnormal areas to become visible. The observer looks at the cervix through the camera and moves it back and forth until the image is in focus. When the image is sharp a picture is taken by pressing a button on the handle.

On the front of the camera is a halogen light source which illuminates the cervix, and a ring flash eliminates shadows from the picture. As the depth of field is nearly five centimetres, it ensures that the whole cervix and some of the surrounding tissue is in focus. A databack on the rear of camera prints a new number on each frame for easy reference later. The photographs can show the presence of abnormal areas on the cervix.

The advantage of cervicography, compared to colposcopy performed by a specialist, is that it can be used in the absence of skilled personnel and performed by medical or paramedical staff such as doctors or nurses who need not be gynaecological specialists. Health workers in family planning centres, for example, could send batches of pictures off for analysis by specialists to detect for any abnormalities and the patient can then be recalled for colposcopy, biopsy, and treatment at the same time if the findings suggest this is necessary. The degree of accuracy is high.

The limitation of the technique includes the difficulty of photographing abnormalities in the cervical canal which may pass undetected by cervicography. But the presence of these could be suspected either by seeing part of the abnormality, visible outside the cervical canal, or by presence of abnormal smear cells and absence of abnormal areas on the cervix. Another disadvantage is that if there is anything to cause suspicion on the cervicograph picture, the patient may be called in for further colposcopic investigation, although no abnormality is to be seen. The disadvantage of having some false positives is obviously preferable to getting a false-negative which is more likely when using cervical smears alone.

How accurate is cervicography?

The indications are that cervicography might be more effective in picking up abnormalities than cervical smears. In a British study by Dr Mike Campion at the Royal Northern Hospital in London, 200 women attending a genito-urinary clinic were examined. Cervicography picked up 98 per cent of the abnormalities of which 58 per cent were not picked up on a smear. The results were backed up by doctors in the US who studied 3000 patients attending for a routine annual smear who also underwent cervicography; 54 of the photographs were classified as abnormal compared with only 12 smears. This suggests that cervicography is more effective at detecting abnormalities.

Thus cervicography should improve and increase the rate of detection and act as a useful ancilliary tool for a colposcopist, or used in the absence of a colposcopist. However, colposcopy is essential in order to take biopsies, establish the diagnosis, and recommend correct treatment.

The introduction of cervicography, particularly in general practice, is likely to increase the number of referrals to colposcopy clinics for biopsy and treatment of abnormal areas, thus putting an even greater strain on an already overloaded service.

Combining cytology, colposcopy and histology

The cytologist, colposcopist and histologist need as much information as possible regarding all the previous smears, colposcopies and biopsies, together with a full and relevant case history of their patient because this extended spectrum of information will give a better basis for any action, treatment and follow-up which is needed. It has been shown that if cytology is used alone, it may miss 2 to 30 per cent of all abnormal cases. Colposcopy, if used alone, without cytology or histology may miss up to 18 per cent of abnormal cases.

Where cytological and histological findings match, then a smear reporting mildly dyskaryotic cells will correspond to CIN 1 (sometimes known as Class 3 smear), moderate dyskaryosis will correspond to CIN 2 (Class 4), severe dyskaryosis to CIN 3 (Class 5). The likelihood of such matching correspondence may not hold true for other smears which may not show a more severe abnormality, subsequently found on histology. For example, doctors at Ninewells Hospital in Dundee studied 228 women with mildly atypical cervical smears who attended the hospital's colposcopy clinic over a ten year period (E.M. Walker *et al.*, *Lancet*, 1986 volume 2, p. 672). 187 women were shown to have mildly dyskaryotic smears and of these, diagnosis of the subsequent biopsies showed that 29.4 per cent had CIN 2 and 39 per cent had CIN 3. 29.2 per cent of the 41 women without dyskaryosis had CIN 2 or 3. Furthermore, 27.6 per cent of the women who had a smear at the time of colposcopy had normal cytology although histology showed a third of these women to have CIN 2 or 3. This suggests that women who have had an atypical smear should always have colposcopy, whether or not a follow-up smear is normal.

The more severe the smear report, the more likely it is to correspond to the histological finding on the biopsy. The more severe the degree of change, the less likely it is to revert to normal and the greater the risk of progression to cancer unless the cells are removed from the body. However, in order to cure a disease it is necessary to know that it exists, hence the need for the cervical smear and subsequent investigations where necessary.

Accuracy of combined investigations

A combination of cytology, colposcopy, histology and a consideration of patients case histories can increase screening accuracy to approximately 98 per cent (compared to around 70 per cent when cytology is used alone) and allows for informed and improved recommendation concerning action and choice of treatment.

In examining both smears and biopsies, cytologists and pathologists may differ between themselves in how they judge a particular sample. What might be a mild abnormality to one person might be interpreted as more advanced by another. In cases where opinions differ, cytology combined with histology is more likely to arrive at the correct diagnosis of a more advanced disease. However, the smear may have failed to pick up any abnormal cells or may have collected cells which show a milder abnormality than actually exists, which is why normal or mildly abnormal smears are sometimes an underestimate of the state of the

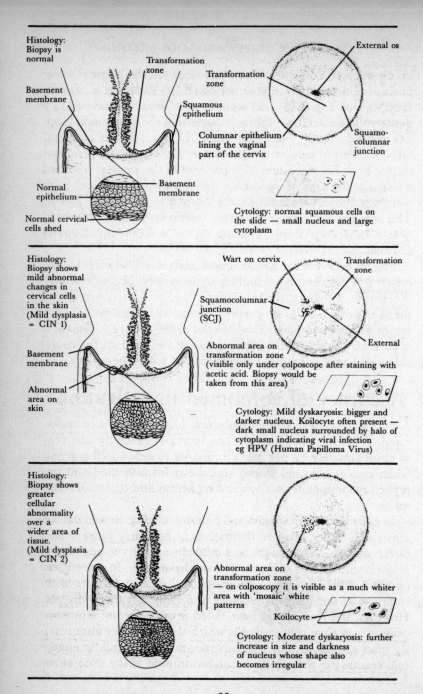

Histology: Biopsy is normal

Transformation zone

Basement membrane

Squamous epithelium

External os

Transformation zone

Columnar epithelium lining the vaginal part of the cervix

Squamo-columnar junction

Normal epithelium

Basement membrane

Normal cervical cells shed

Cytology: normal squamous cells on the slide — small nucleus and large cytoplasm

Histology: Biopsy shows mild abnormal changes in cervical cells in the skin (Mild dysplasia = CIN 1)

Wart on cervix

Transformation zone

Squamocolumnar junction (SCJ)

Basement membrane

External

Abnormal area on transformation zone (visible only under colposcope after staining with acetic acid. Biopsy would be taken from this area)

Abnormal area on skin

Cytology: Mild dyskaryosis: bigger and darker nucleus. Koilocyte often present — dark small nucleus surrounded by halo of cytoplasm indicating viral infection eg HPV (Human Papilloma Virus)

Histology: Biopsy shows greater cellular abnormality over a wider area of tissue. (Mild dysplasia = CIN 2)

Abnormal area on transformation zone — on colposcopy it is visible as a much whiter area with 'mosaic' white patterns

Koilocyte

Cytology: Moderate dyskaryosis: further increase in size and darkness of nucleus whose shape also becomes irregular

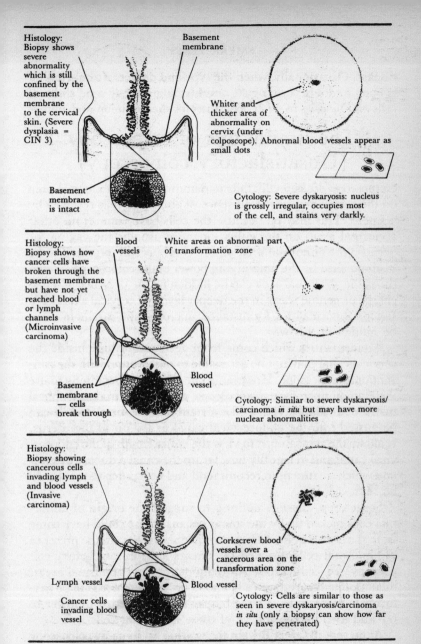

Histology: Biopsy shows severe abnormality which is still confined by the basement membrane to the cervical skin. (Severe dysplasia = CIN 3)

Basement membrane

Basement membrane is intact

Whiter and thicker area of abnormality on cervix (under colposcope). Abnormal blood vessels appear as small dots

Cytology: Severe dyskaryosis: nucleus is grossly irregular, occupies most of the cell, and stains very darkly.

Histology: Biopsy shows how cancer cells have broken through the basement membrane but have not yet reached blood or lymph channels (Microinvasive carcinoma)

Blood vessels

White areas on abnormal part of transformation zone

Basement membrane — cells break through

Blood vessel

Cytology: Similar to severe dyskaryosis/carcinoma in situ but may have more nuclear abnormalities

Histology: Biopsy showing cancerous cells invading lymph and blood vessels (Invasive carcinoma)

Corkscrew blood vessels over a cancerous area on the transformation zone

Lymph vessel

Cancer cells invading blood vessel

Blood vessel

Cytology: Cells are similar to those as seen in severe dyskaryosis/carcinoma in situ (only a biopsy can show how far they have penetrated)

Figure 8 The cytological and histological differences between a normal, pre-cancerous and cancerous cervix.

disease. Occasionally, when the type and degree of abnormality is open to doubt, cytologists and histologists may send slides of cells and biopsies to other specialists for their opinion and advice.

The limitations of colposcopy (Unsatisfactory colposcopy)

Colposcopy occasionally fails to demonstrate an abnormal area on the cervix despite the presence of abnormal cells revealed by a smear. This may be because the cells have come from other abnormal areas on the vulva, or more usually, the vagina, or because the abnormal area on the cervix is still too small to be distinguished by the magnifying power of the colposcope. Sometimes the abnormal area can be hidden by the presence of a discharge or genital warts in the deeper layers of cervical skin. Very serious abnormalities, for instance, microinvasive carcinoma, can be hidden in this way.

Abnormalities which come from deep and/or high inside the cervical canal may not be accessible to observation with the conventional colposcope. However, some clinics are beginning to use the Hamou microhysterocolposcope, a recently introduced optical instrument shaped rather like a rigid narrow metal rod. It can be passed into the endocervical canal as far up as the uterus. It allows the colposcopist to view the entire length of the endocervical canal and to identify how far up the canal a disease extends and which treatment to recommend and how much tissue should be removed.

Sometimes, there is nothing to suggest the origin of abnormal cells picked up by the smear because these could have come from the uterus or even from the Fallopian tubes. In the presence of abnormal cells revealed by smears and 'unsatisfactory colposcopy', i.e. failing to see or demonstrate any abnormal areas, dilatation and curettage (a D and C or 'scrape') needs to be performed. Sometimes, a cone biopsy may be needed in order to try and identify the source of these malignant cells.

At present in Great Britain the waiting list in many colposcopy clinics for evaluation of an abnormal smear is as much as several months. The increasing number of referrals of women with abnormal smears to hospital colposcopy clinics indicates a vast increase in pre-invasive cervical disease which has already over-stretched existing hospital resources as is shown by the long waiting times for colposcopy and treatment.

Proper training and good quality control is essential to achieve good results with colposcopy (and the same applies to cytology and histology). The scarcity of colposcopy services is due to the fact they are expensive. As well as the cost of the colposcopic equipment, it costs a lot of money to train a doctor into a competent colposcopist as it is a very time-consuming process. Colposcopists are not purely technicians, they are also diagnosticians. Before they can recommend treatment, they must consider not only the cytology, colposcopic findings and subsequent histological report, but also the case history and the age of the patient concerned and the availability of future follow-up screening. It is often the colposcopist who recommends the treatment and, if the experience of the colposcopist were to be inadequate, local treatment of the cervical skin might subsequently be found to have been inadequate and inappropriate because a more deeply seated pre-cancer or invasive cancer has been missed. Local treatment will not remove the deeper lying invasive cancer which can continue to progress undetected, particularly if the patient does not attend for follow-up smears.

Chapter 5

Treatment of cervical pre-cancer (CIN)

- CIN can be treated locally (i.e. physical removal of the entire abnormal tissue without removal of the cervix). Treatment involves removing the abnormal tissue by one of the following: cryocautery; electrodiathermy or 'cold' coagulation; laser evaporation; or excision.

- Local treatments are usually very successful in eradicating the disease whilst at the same time preserving the structure and function of the cervix.

- A cone biopsy is required for any CIN which cannot be seen in its entirety under colposcopy or where the biopsy suggests a possibility of microinvasion. This diagnostic technique removes a larger piece of cervical tissue than the local treatments. If the abnormality is fully contained within the cone biopsy then treatment is complete. If it extends beyond the cone margin, hysterectomy may be required.

- Follow-up colposcopy and smears within a year, and preferably after four months of initial treatment, are essential.

- Annual smears are recommended for all women who have undergone treatment for CIN as it may re-occur after treatment. Re-treatment may then be necessary.

In order to be completely successful, treatment aims to remove all the abnormal pre-cancerous or cancerous cells from the body.

If this is not done, then any abnormal cells that are left behind, will continue to grow and multiply, and may spread and invade and ultimately kill the patient. As well as removing the abnormality, the treatment also aims to preserve remaining healthy tissue and to cause a minimum of damage and discomfort to the patient. At present, no drug exists which will effectively kill pre-cancer or cancer cells completely without having serious adverse effects on the rest of the body.

Before accurate information from cytology and, later, colposcopy and histology, became available regarding the presence, nature, and depth of penetration by abnormal cells, treatment was usually late and mainly by cone biopsy or hysterectomy.

While these methods of treatment were successful in removing the disease, providing it had not spread beyond the confines of the tissue removed, they were often too radical, in that major surgery was often performed to remove a very minor abnormality. Thus patients were subjected to major operations which carried their own risk of mortality and morbidity and often deprived women of their reproductive functions.

Today, we have cytology, colposcopy and histology. These techniques, coupled with a knowledge of the patient and good clinical examination, allow for a good and reasonably accurate assessment regarding the nature and extent of cervical disease. This information can now be used in the choice of one of a number of highly effective treatments which can be tailored to destroy only the area of diseased tissue—minimal treatment providing a cure and preventing a potentially major illness.

Recent advances in medical technology have placed a wide variety of useful instruments with which to perform such treatments at doctors' disposal, and there is the prospect of even more sophisticated diagnostic and curative methods in the future.

Local treatments of CIN

When the abnormal area is completely visible under the colposcope and the biopsy reveals that the cells have not invaded or penetrated too deeply, it is possible to remove the entire affected area by a local ablative treatment, abbreviated to LAT. This is done by methods which will be described shortly. A new skin grows over the cervix after treatment to leave a healthy region and the patient is considered cured from the disease. Because it is the transformation zone in which pre-cancerous changes tend to be initially induced, treatment aims to remove not only the affected area of abnormality but also to destroy the entire transformation zone. It is thus reasonable to expect that by removing this area in its entirety, one can remove a prospective breeding ground for infection and reduce the likelihood of pre-cancer reoccurring.

Assessment and choice of treatment depends on the combined results of cytology, colposcopy and histology, coupled with a knowledge of a patient's case history and a good clinical examination. The results of a smear may act as a warning sign indicating the existence of abnormal cells; colposcopy defines the size and extent of abnormal areas on the cervix; and histology indicates the degree of abnormality and depth of penetration and presence or absence of invasion beyond the cervical skin.

The types of treatment available today allow precise areas of abnormality to be eradicated completely with minimal damage to surrounding tissues and such treatment can be confirmed visually by colposcopy and histology. However, ten to fifteen years ago the situation was very different because techniques did not exist to define the size and extent of the abnormality suggested by cytological results from smears. In an attempt to remove the diseased area, a variable sized cone-shaped piece of tissue was removed (cone biopsy) from the cervix. Cone biopsy usually removes the entire transformation zone and the area up to the internal os. This was then examined histologically to discover whether all the abnormality had been removed. Cone biopsy often removed a lot of normal tissue unecessarily along with the abnormal tissue and sometimes damaged the cervix. The cone biopsy combined diagnosis and treatment in one procedure. This method is still employed when the abnormal area cannot be completely defined by colposcopy. It is also performed when the smear suggests a far greater abnormality than can be seen on either colposcopy or histology, or where colposcopy is not available.

In Britain and the United States, conization was initially used as a diagnostic procedure to identify the amount of invasion by the cancer. In other European countries and Scandinavia, conization was performed after colposcopic evaluation and used as a therapeutic procedure. After colposcopy became more widely available in the English-speaking countries, conization became the treatment of choice and was used in some cases where previously hysterectomy may have been performed to ensure the removal of the disease. Conization is an excellent treatment for CIN, but there are several reasons why it may be unsatisfactory or indeed unnecessary.

Firstly, conization was, and may still be followed by several days in hospital as an in-patient which means cost for the health service and also to the patient who may have to spend time off work. Secondly, the operation carries a risk of possible haemorrhage or infection. Thirdly, stenosis may occur which makes it difficult to obtain either satisfactory smears or adequate colposcopic assessment in the future. Stenosis can cause painful periods and difficulty in opening the cervix during labour which may make Caesarean section necessary. Conversely, a cone biopsy may leave the cervix in a lax state in which a pregnancy cannot be retained in the uterus satisfactorily, resulting in miscarriage or premature delivery.

One of the reasons why it is very important to remove precancerous cells by more conservative methods than cone biopsy is the dramatic rise in the rate of cervical pre-cancer in the last five years affecting young women. Many of them have never had children and most of them are anxious to maintain their reproductive potential. Conization does present a threat to their fertility, although more than 90 per cent of women will go on to have a normal pregnancy following conization. In recent years, new treatments have been developed which remove only the abnormal tissue with minimal damage to surrounding areas. This is far less traumatic and has fewer of the problems associated with conization mentioned above. The development of these new techniques came in parallel with improved cervical examination.

By using colposcopy and biopsy, new local treatments other than cone biopsy can be carried out effectively. Such treatments involve physical removal of abnormal skin to the depth or extent indicated by the histology of the cervical biopsy. We have already discussed the use of cone biopsy which may act as both a diagnostic tool and a form of treatment if the biopsy eradicates the whole of an abnormal area. In more than 99 per cent of cases the abnormality will have been eradicated using this treatment.

Local ablative treatment (LAT)

There are several destructive local techniques which can be directed precisely at the diseased tissue.

They include:

- Cryocautery—freezing
- Electrodiathermy—burning
- Cold coagulation—boiling
- Laser evaporation or excision—use of laser energy
- Loop excision (LLETZ)

Before a doctor goes ahead with local removal of the abnormal area there must be no question of any invasive cancer. If any abnormal cells remain deep under the area being treated, they will continue to invade deeper into tissues. At one time it was feared that the new skin which grew over the malignant cells masked their existence and thus prevented detection on future smears or by colposcopy. However it has been shown recently that the pre-cancerous cells are shed as before and can still be detected on smears.

If there is an existing pelvic infection this should always be treated first because it may complicate both local or general treatment by flaring up afterwards or increase the likelihood of bleeding after treatment and of delaying healing.

Cryocautery

Cryocautery (also known as cryosurgery or cryotherapy) is performed on an out-patient basis with little discomfort and takes as little as fifteen minutes to complete. A colposcope is used to determine the extent of the diseased area and then a gynaecologist freezes the cervix for a few minutes using carbon dioxide or nitrous oxide delivered with a gun pipe unit with interchangeable probes. It is particularly appropriate for very small, localized and superficial mild changes in the cervix and destruction of the area is only to a depth of 2-5 mm, occasionally up to 8 mm. It is relatively painless, needs no anaesthesia, side-effects are minor and include faintness and mild abdominal cramp during the procedure and a watery discharge for two or three weeks after treatment.

The effectiveness of cryocautery treatment for CIN varies depending on the severity and area of CIN. At best it should be recommended for small CIN 1 or CIN 2 lesions. A problem it may create is that the endocervix tends to be tightened after such treatment making subsequent smears difficult.

The success rate for eradicating the disease at the first treatment is 80-90 per cent. Follow-up smears and colpsocopy within six months are needed to confirm whether the treatment has been successful. Cryocautery may be repeated if necessary.

Cryocautery is only suitable for small areas of abnormality and where the disease is CIN 1 or 2, although sometimes it is used for CIN 3.

Diathermy or electrocoagulation

This involves the destruction of the abnormal area using electrically generated heat applied through needle and ball electrodes and the entire abnormal area is destroyed by burning. The depth of destruction is determined by the operator. Diathermy is highly effective in eradicating all varieties of CIN and up to 97 per cent of patients who have had abnormal areas removed by diathermy needed only a single treatment. The other three per cent may have needed a second treatment. Because it is a painful procedure, a general anaesthetic is needed, which necessitates a stay in hospital.

During the burning of the abnormal tissue it is unavoidable that some of the neighbouring normal tissue is also damaged. This results in a prolonged bloody discharge lasting two or three weeks after treatment, during which sexual intercourse should be avoided to reduce the risk of infection. Occasionally, healing is delayed. There is an increased risk of stenosis of the cervical canal and, depending on how tight it becomes, it may make it difficult to obtain future adequate cervical smears or satisfactory colposcopy assessment. Sometimes the flow of menstrual discharge is also obstructed and this may cause painful periods and it may be necessary to dilate the cervix. However, the very high rate of permanent eradication with only one treatment makes diathermy a very useful treatment.

Diathermy loop excision (see also p.74)

Loop excision of CIN from the cervix is becoming more and more popular as an ablative treatment. The advantage of this treatment compared to others such as cone biopsy or laser, is that it is cheap, can be performed at the same time as a colposcopic examination, and preserves the tissue — usually the whole transformation zone — which is removed for histological examination to ensure the CIN has been removed in its entirety.

Cold coagulation

This simple, cheap and effective treatment involves the application of a probe to the cervix through which heat is generated and the abnormal area is destroyed, usually in less than two minutes. This technique has few significant side effects, although heavy discharge and some destruction of normal healthy tissue surrounding the area may occur (as it can with diathermy). The advantage of this method is that general anaesthesia is not required and a 95 per cent cure rate for CIN 3 lesion using cold coagulation is reported.

It might seem peculiar to call it 'cold' coagulation when the temperature is usually at 100° Centigrade, but this is much cooler than the very high temperature (up to 1000°C) used in diathermy.

Laser treatment

In colposcopic clinics, lasers are used to provide a source of energy either to evaporate diseased tissue or cut around and remove a piece of abnormal area for histological examination.

History

Lasers were first used for the treatment of CIN in the United States as recently as 1974 and the first laser used in Britain was introduced into the Birmingham and Midlands Hospital for Women in August 1977. In the beginning, the results obtained were extremely poor, with a large proportion of patients having residual abnormality following a single laser evaporation. This was explained by the fact that the tissue was not destroyed to a great enough depth. By trial and error, it has been shown that laser depth of destruction should aim to be at least 7mm. This technique results in a very clean and effective destruction of the CIN.

If the laser is used only for vaporization, the entire affected area and the whole of the transformation zone on the cervix will be evaporated into thin air and will not be available for future histological reference. It is possible to use laser for cutting out and thus preserving abnormal tissues. Either evaporation or cutting of the cervix by laser produces very little pain. Different people experience pain differently when they are being treated. To prevent discomfort, a local anaesthetic may be injected with a very fine syringe directly and painlessly into the cervix. Because the laser beam has a very small diameter it is possible to remove or destroy the diseased area with minimal damage to the neighbouring tissues. Also, the laser beam seals the local tissues, including blood vessels, thereby preventing bleeding.

As with any destructive technique the following criteria have to be met before this sort of treatment can be considered. The patient has to be seen and assessed by a colposcopist who examines the entire diseased area; the possibility of invasive carcinoma must have been excluded. The need for good cytological and colposcopic follow-up for the future continues. The treatment should be avoided during a period or pregnancy.

The advantage of laser treatment is that in up to 70 per cent of cases where the CIN is visible, it can be removed without any form of anaesthesia on an out-patient basis. General anaesthesia may be required when the area to be destroyed is very large and its destruction may take some time, thus generating heat and pain. Some women are very sensitive to even minor injury to the cervix and, to avoid this pain, they may want a general anaesthetic. If the laser is being used to remove vulvo-vaginal warts at the same time, this also necessitates general anaesthesia. Healing begins almost immediately after treatment and a new disease-free lining grows, and this lining is less susceptible to CIN.

Problems after laser treatment

More than 95 per cent of patients subjected to laser treatment experience no problems at all. Occasionally, bleeding may occur during the treatment but it is not usually a problem. In around 1.5 per cent of patients bleeding occurs within a few days of treatment and can be stopped by the application of silver nitrate sticks. The cervix heals rapidly following laser treatment and appears healed within four weeks. The only drawback is that intercourse should be avoided, as it should following all the other types of treatment, for up to four to six weeks after treatment.

Laser treatment is highly effective. Around 95 per cent of patients treated remain free from the disease for the first year after treatment. However, some cases do reoccur and patients are advised to have annual smears in years to come and to have re-treatment where necessary. Lasers can also be used to perform cone biopsies. The advantage of this, compared to using a conventional scalpel, is that the heat of the beam causes coagulation of the local blood vessels, which reduces bleeding. Stitching is usually unnecessary.

Laser treatment does not impair fertility or future delivery of a baby except where successive treatments of a reoccurring pre-cancer has diminished the volume of cervical tissue to such an extent that the holding capability of the cervix has been reduced.

Which treatment?

Choice of treatment depends on colposcopic and histological findings and on a patient's individual circumstances. We have described which treatments are appropriate for which conditions, but often the reality is that you get what is available. For example, small hospitals cannot afford lasers, so they will use whatever method is available. Fortunately, since the spread of colposcopy, local treatments can be accurately targeted onto the diseased pre-cancerous tissue and the success rate with all the local removals is very high.

Follow-ups

The importance of follow-up examinations after treatment is to ensure the disease has been removed and that there are no side-effects resulting from treatment. Whilst most local treatments are highly successful, it is not possible to guarantee a cure or remove the possibility of recurrence. It is possible that the process which initiated the original disease may still exist and therefore it is essential to have follow-up attendances during which smears, with or without colposcopy, are needed to detect the presence of abnormality.

Follow-ups should take place within a year, and preferably four to six months after treatment. Ideally, a smear should be combined with colposcopy. A smear alone may sometimes miss the disease, particularly as the cervix may have become stenosed. After the first year, smears should be taken annually whether the patient continues to have sexual intercourse or not.

Recurrence and local re-treatment

The disease may reoccur following treatment either because treatment failed to remove the disease completely, or because it is a completely new occurrence. Treatment is the same as for the original incidence of the disease. Re-treatment is usually very succesful. Since the local treatment removes a definite volume of the cervical tissue, it follows that at each re-treatment, a further diminution of cervical tissue will take place.

Table 7 Comparison of local conservative methods of destruction of CIN

	Cone biopsy	Diathermy*
Technique	Removal of cone of cervical tissue using a knife or laser	Burning away tissue by applying a diathermy ball to the cervix
Anaesthesia	General with a knife. Local with a laser	General
Accuracy of destruction	Available from histology report	Approx.
Destruction depth	Variable known from histology report	Approx. 5-10mm
Treatment	Up to 1 hour	Up to half an hour
Time in hospital	In-patient 3-4 days (Usually out-patient for laser)	In-patient 1-3 days
Discharge	Moderate/ heavy 3-4 weeks	Heavy 14-20 days
Healing time	Approx. 6 weeks	Approx. 4 weeks
Pain	Severe for few days	Moderate for few days
Cure rate	<92%	<93%
Haemorrhage	Occasional	Less frequent
Stenosis	Occasional	Very occasional
Pregnancy Delivery	Problems sometimes	Very rarely any problems
Future smear sampling	May be difficult	Problems may occur if cervix is stenosed

* Diathermy loop excision technique described on page 74. The other criteria are similar to those described for laser treatment on page 97.

TREATMENT OF CERVICAL PRE-CANCER

Cryocautery	Laser	Cold coagulation
Freezing of tissue by carbon dioxide or nitrous oxide	Evaporation or cutting out of tissue with laser beam which emits electro-magnetic radiation of high intensity	Burning of cervix with heated Teflon probe
None	Local	Local
Approx.	Within 1mm if tissue cut out for histology	Approx.
Approx. 2-3mm	Up to 10mm	7 to 10 mm
Up to half an hour	Up to 10 mins	Up to 10 mins
Out-patient	Out-patient	Out-patient
Moderate 14-28 days	Light 7-14 days	Light 7-14 days
Approx. 4-5 weeks	Approx. Under 3 weeks	Up to three weeks
Slight discomfort felt only at treatment	Occasional mild discomfort at treatment	Occasional mild discomforts
<80-95%	>93%	95%
Rare	Rare—easily stopped	Very rare—stopped easily
Rare	Rare	Rare
Unaffected	Unaffected	Unaffected
Very occasional problems	Usually problem-free	Usually problem-free

Chapter 6

Invasive cervical cancer

- If CIN 3 or carcinoma *in situ* is left untreated, 20-30 per cent of cases will progress to invasive cancer. The rate of progress is at present unpredictable, and it is not possible to identify which CINs will progress. In order to prevent any progression it is advisable to remove CIN in its entirety.

- Invasive cancer occurs when the cancerous cells have penetrated beyond the basement membrane of the cervix.

- Around 90 per cent of invasive cancers will develop signs or symptoms such as irregular bleeding, discharges and abdominal and pelvic pains.

- The disease is classified under a 'staging' system which takes account of which nearby organs and vessels have been invaded.

- Staging provides a surgeon with a guide to appropriate treatment.

- Physical examinations, lymphograms, intravenous urograms, ultrasound, CAT scans, and NMR can be used to identify the stage and existence and spread of invasive cancers.

If CIN 3 or carcinoma *in situ* pass undetected, some 20-30 per cent of them will progress into invasive cancer. It is not possible to predict the speed with which these changes will occur. Invasive cervical cancer occurs when the cancerous cells have not only penetrated and broken through the deepest layer of the skin known as the basement membrane on which the skin rests, but may also have entered the lymphatic and blood channels.

Staging cervical cancer

In the same way that histologists use the term 'CIN' to describe the degree of abnormality within the cervical skin, the penetration, extent and metastasis of invasive cancer in the body are described in terms of *staging*. The first 'stage' in this progression is known as 'microinvasive disease' where the CIN 3 has broken through the basement membrane of the cervical skin, but is no more than 3mm through the epithelial base, and has not yet entered the lymphatic channels which would spread it into other organs. This is known as Stage I*a* under the staging system of the International Federation of Obstetrics and Gynaecology.

A more advanced form of invasion is known as **occult invasive carcinoma** Stage I*b*, where there may be no clinical symptoms, but where invasion is more than 3mm from the epithelial base. The lymphatic channels may be involved. If the lymphatic channels are involved the cancer may spread whatever the treatment.

Table 8 **Staging classification of cervical pre-cancer and cancer**

Stage 0	(CIN 3 [carcinoma *in situ*]) cancer is still confined to cervical skin
Stage I*a*	(Microinvasive carcinoma) Cancerous cells have broken through basement membrane but not entered lymphatic or blood channels
Stage I*b*	(Occult invasive carcinoma) Cancerous cells have broken through to beyond 3mm from basement membrane and the lymphatic channels may be involved
Stage II*a*	Invasion into part of the vagina
Stage II*b*	Invasion into tissue around the cervix
Stage III	Invasion into lower vagina and pelvic wall
Stage IV	Invasion beyond genital area into nearby organs.

In Stage I, there is a clearly definable cancer which is confined to the cervix and can be seen with a colposcope. If the cancer has spread beyond the cervix, but not onto the pelvic wall, this is known as Stage II which can be subdivided into II*a* and II*b*. Stage II*a* includes invasion of the upper part of the vagina, and Stage IIb describes invasion into the tissues surrounding the uterus (the parametrium).

When the cancer spreads into the pelvic wall and the lower third of the vagina it is referred to as Stage III, and if it spreads more widely into the bladder, and rectum, it is known as Stage IV.

The importance and necessity of staging is to give the surgeon adequate information on where the disease is and how much tissue should be removed. If the extent of the disease is underestimated, the removal of affected tissue will be incomplete and the disease will continue to progress.

Stage 0, 1*a* and 1*b* can be determined using cytology, punch biopsy and cone biopsy. During these stages there are rarely any obvious symptoms although there may be bleeding after intercourse or at times other than menstruation. Where there is any suspicion of further involvement, such as that provided by biopsy, clinical examination, and patient symptoms, further investigations are needed in order to discover how far the disease has spread.

Identifying cancerous growths

Signs and Symptoms

There are a number of signs and symptoms which may point to the existence and nature of the disease.

Once the cancer has spread beyond the basement membrane, almost 90 per cent of invasive carcinoma cases are of a clinically recognizable type, with the earliest signs being bleeding, which may initially be irregular and brought on by sexual intercourse, or may become apparent after passing urine or on opening one's bowels. As the cancer becomes more invasive, the bleeding may persist in varying quantity. As the growth ulcerates and becomes infected, there may be an offensive smelling and thin blood-stained discharge. Painful symptoms such as backache may indicate that the cancer has spread beyond the cervix. In advanced cases of invasion the bleeding may be very heavy, the discharge copious and extremely foul smelling. Lower abdominal pain may result from the growth of a large pelvic mass or in the lower back if there is an extension of tumour into the uterosacral ligaments (the supporting ligaments of the uterus).

Very severe and intractable pain may result from involvement of lymph nodes which have adhered to the sacral plexus (the network of nerve fibres in the pelvis). Presence of malignant cells in the pelvic bones may also cause back pain.

In the very late stages, there may be single or double incontinence (inability to control the bladder and bowel) as ulceration may continue into the bladder and rectum. The patient is in constant distress and loses weight. Sepsis and pain are also important contributory factors. Death is most commonly due to uraemia (build-up of toxins in the blood) following the blockage of both ureters (the ducts which convey urine from the kidney to the bladder) or to ascending pyelonephritis (infection affecting the kidney), but it sometimes occurs from haemorrhage or the effects of metastases.

Physical examination

The doctor can feel for the presence of masses on the cervix, vagina, or pelvis. Examination under anaesthetic (EUA) can improve the physical examination as it relaxes the abdominal muscles, thereby facilitating examination of the whole genital region. The cervical canal may be widened (dilatation) so that a small instrument is inserted into the uterus and the lining of the uterus scraped out (curettage) for examination. The whole process is commonly referred to as a 'D and C', i.e. dilatation and curettage. D and C is a standard and routine gynaecological procedure for obtaining tissues from the uterus and endocervix for laboratory examination. If indicated, the bladder and rectum may also be viewed by cystoscopy (inspection of the bladder) and proctoscopy (inspection of the rectum) respectively.

Other investigative techniques

If there is an indication that the cancer may have spread into the lymphatic channels, glands and other parts of the body, then further investigations are needed so that appropriate surgical treatment can be recommended.

Intravenous urogram

As the local spread of cancer may involve parts of the urinary system, which includes kidneys, ureters, bladder, and urethra, it may be useful to investigate them using an **intravenous urogram** (IVU). Most patients suspected of having the invasive disease will have an IVU. This involves injecting a radio-opaque (i.e. it shows up on X-ray) dye into a vein in the arm. This dye is concentrated in the urinary system where the X-ray pictures taken may detect tumours.

Lymphogram

This technique involves X-raying the abdomen and pelvis to identify those lymph nodes in which tumour cells have lodged. Special radio-opaque dye is injected via lymph channels in the feet from where it spreads, outlining the lymph glands in the pelvis and around the cervical region, and highlights the presence of tumours which would not be visible otherwise. Bluish-green urine for the next day or so is a common after-effect of this technique caused by the dye being excreted.

CAT scan (Computerized Axial Tomography)

On rare occasions, a woman may be offered a CAT scan if such facilities exist in her area. Such scans are performed in hospital and involve taking X-rays at different positions so that a computer can build up a two and three dimensional image of the body. An hour and also again thirty minutes before a scan, one is asked to drink a radio-opaque liquid which allows the abnormalities to be easily detected on X-ray. The vagina is normally opened slightly by the insertion of a tampon prior to the scan.

NMR (Nuclear magnetic resonance)

A few women may also be offered an NMR scan. This involves subjecting the patient to strong magnetic waves which react in a different way when passing through tumours than they do when passing through normal tissues. These differences are shown on computer-generated television images. NMR is preferable to CAT scanning because it does not involve the use of radiation. However, the cost and running of NMR machinery has so far restricted it to a very few hospitals. Another problems associated with NMR, and also CAT scans, is that these techniques cannot identify tumours less than two centimetres in diameter.

Ultrasound scan

In a few cases, an ultrasound scan may be offered. This technique involves the use of sound waves which can travel through the body, and measure the degree of reflection, which depends on the type of structures they hit. This reflection can be translated into a television image for analysis. Ultrasound is not as accurate and reliable as CAT and NMR, but is widely available, very safe, and takes less than half an hour. It involves a gel being applied to the abdomen and a small probe run backwards and forwards through the gel, bouncing sound waves through the body.

In the methods described above, tumours appear differently from normal tissues, and an idea of the presence, size, and extent of the cancerous growth can be obtained. However, it may be necessary to use a combination of these techniques as no single investigation is ever absolutely reliable.

The limitation of all these techniques is that, although they detect cancer after it has reached certain dimensions, they may fail to detect single abnormal cells which have the potential to travel around the body and subsequently give rise to further tumours. This explains why treatment which initially appears complete may have failed to eradicate the disease.

Chapter 7

Treatment of microinvasive and invasive cancer

- Microinvasive carcinoma up to a depth of 3mm can be treated by cone biopsy. If it extends deeper, hysterectomy may be needed.

- Early invasive cancer (Stage 1*b* and II*a*) is treated by hysterectomy.

- An ovary may be left in place in young women to help maintain their hormone levels.

- Radiotherapy may be used to treat some patients, particularly those who may be unsuitable for surgery, such as elderly patients.

- Radiotherapy is usually used to treat advanced forms of cervical cancer.

- Exenteration (extensive removal of organs within the pelvis) may be necessary if the disease re-occurs.

- Length of survival depends on the severity and spread of the disease and also on its correct staging, thus enabling identification and removal of cancerous tissue.

- One or two women in every thousand who have a smear will have an invasive cancer. Of those women who have a positive smear, around one in three hundred will have an invasive cancer.

Microinvasive carcinoma
This is where the disease has penetrated to a depth of up to 3 millimetres beneath the basement membrane but has not invaded the lymph nodes. It is treated either by conization or hysterectomy.

Invasive carcinoma
This is where cancerous cells have broken beyond 3mm from the basement membrane (the layer of tissue which divides the cervical skin from underlying tissues where blood vessels and lymphatics are found). The cells may have entered the blood stream or lymphatic channels and spread beyond the cervix.

Fortunately, of every thousand women who have a smear, only one or two will have invasive carcinoma, and, of those who have a positive smear, only one in three hundred will be shown to have an invasive cancer.

History

Until the beginning of the twentieth century cervical cancer was considered incurable. Death within two years was common and usually involved tremendous suffering. At the beginning of this century, a Viennese doctor called Ernst Wertheim, who had looked closely at autopsy material from women who had suffered cervical cancer, designed a surgical procedure which removed the uterus (hysterectomy) and surrounding lymph glands. Of the first hundred patients which Wertheim operated on, thirty died as a result of the operation.

While Wertheim and others were pioneers in the surgical treatment of invasive cancer, the Curies were demonstrating the effects of radiation. An institute in Stockholm opened for the radiation treatment of patients with cancer. The first radiation 'cure' of cervical cancer was in 1911. Radiation treatment subsequently became more popular and surgery was condemned to take a back seat. Medical students were taught that the treatment for cervical cancer was by radiation and surgical procedures were not to be used. However, radiation only cured around 40 per cent of cases. Today, it is common for radiation treatment to be used in combination with surgery. For example, radiation may be used to sterilize infected tumours prior to surgery.

Treating microinvasive carcinoma

Microinvasive carcinoma is treated either by conization or hysterectomy. Conization (cone biopsy) is preferred when the disease is identified in young women who still want children. Conization is performed when the microinvasion does not extend beyond three millimeteres beneath the basement membrane. If it goes further, then a hysterectomy may be necessary whatever the age of the patient.

Some doctors recommend hysterectomy for a microinvasive carcinoma which is less than three millimetres if a woman does not want children or is beyond child-bearing age. Attitudes have changed from a 'hysterectomy for all' view to one of selective conization where possible. The latter approach requires diligent follow-up to ensure that the patient remains free of cancer.

Treating early invasive cancer

Surgery

Once invasive cancer has spread, the average time from the onset of symptoms to death is about two years if the disease is left untreated. In the early stages of invasive cancer when the disease is confined to the womb (Stage Ib), or has encroached into the top of the vagina (Stage IIa), a radical hysterectomy (which includes removing the Fallopian tubes, ovaries and lymph nodes as well as the uterus and cervix) may be recommended. The operation is performed under general anaesthesia.

Ovarian hormones influence the state of the linings of the genital tract and help to preserve the density of the bone. Removal of ovaries before menopause induces a 'surgical' menopause with side effects such as hot flushes, feelings of general exhaustion and loss of sexual drive. Ovaries are removed in older women in order to diminish the risk of potential ovarian cancer which may occur in this age group. In this instance, the loss of ovarian hormones may require a long term hormone replacement therapy (HRT) in order to counteract hot flushes, bone loss, and atrophy of genital and mucous linings.

Patients can come home one to two weeks after a hysterectomy which is performed in hospital under general anaesthetic.

Depending on the extent of hysterectomy performed and an individual's power of recovery, it can take four to six weeks or even longer to fully recover from such an operation. During this time sexual intercourse and heavy physical work should be avoided. If, at a follow-up appointment with the surgeon after six weeks or so, an internal examination reveals that satisfactory healing has taken place, sex, work, and sport can start again. Although the cervix will have been removed during hysterectomy, it is still important for a woman to have an initial colposcopic examination and annual vaginal smears to ensure the disease has not remained, as could be the case if the abnormality initially extended from the cervix onto the vaginal wall and escaped identification and removal.

Radiotherapy

Radiotherapy may be the treatment of choice, particularly for older patients who are difficult to treat surgically, or patients whose tumours have spread and become difficult to eradicate completely by surgery.

There are two forms of radiotherapy:

Internal radiotherapy

This involves using small tubes or packets containing a radioactive form of metals such as caesium or cobalt, which are inserted into the vagina. The radiation produced is delivered quickly to the cancer and its surrounding tissues. Dosages of radioactivity are determined according to the individual. The treatment involves a doctor inserting the applicator into the vagina so that it is near the cervix. This is performed in a hospital under general anaesthetic and the applicator is usually left in position for less than 24 hours.

External radiotherapy

This involves visiting a hospital radiotherapy unit as an outpatient where a beam of high energy X-rays (gamma rays) is directed at tumours. This is given to cover the possibility of extension of cancerous cells beyond the primary site of the tumour and can be used to irradiate the lymph nodes which if untreated will enable cancerous cells to travel to and lodge in vital organs around the body. Doctors plan correct therapy during visits prior to treatment where a small amount of barium, a liquid which shows up clearly on X-rays, is injected into the rectum. This is to identify the precise location of the tumour site before radiation is administered. Treatment is usually for up to five days a week for between three and six weeks. External radiotherapy may be administered after surgery has removed a tumour.

Side effects of radiotherapy

Tiredness, particularly an hour or two after treatment is a common side effect of radiotherapy. There may also be nausea, although this can be alleviated by medicines, drinking plenty of fluids, and eating little and often, avoiding greasy and highly spiced foods. Alcohol should be avoided. The bowels are likely to be loose for several weeks after treatment. The skin between the groin and buttocks may feel sore, a bit like a sunburn, and daily baths with plain warm water followed by patting dry with a soft towel and application of unscented talcum powder may alleviate discomfort.

A slight burning sensation on passing urine can be eased by drinking plenty of fluids and and also by medication. The vagina may become dry after radiotherapy so a lubricant may be necessary to facilitate sexual intercourse.

Radiation versus surgery

The treatment of Stage I*b* by radiation or surgery has roughly identical results, with around 85 per cent of patients surviving for five years following either treatment. However, survival depends on whether the lymph nodes are involved. If the nodes are clear from any cancerous cells, then there is only around a ten per cent risk of recurrence. But in the 12 per cent of women who have nodal invasion by the malignant cells, their five-year survival can be less than 20 per cent if five or more nodes are involved, or around 50 per cent when one to four nodes have been invaded.

The disadvantage of radiotherapy compared to surgery is that it can cause serious bladder or bowel damage in a small percentage of patients (2-6 per cent), may cause early menopause as a result of irradiation of the ovaries which can be conserved in surgery, and may result in tightening or tissue damage to the vagina and thus lead to painful sex.

Furthermore, the patient recovers more quickly from surgery which is also cheaper than radiotherapy. However, the disadvantage is that there may be surgical complications, especially involving bladder and urinary tract damage.

Some doctors advocate a combination of surgery and radiotherapy, but opinion is divided as to whether the results are better than with either treatment performed alone.

Advanced cervical cancer

For women with Stage II*b*, III, and IV, radiotherapy is usually the treatment of choice. For women with Stage II, the five-year survival outlook is between 45-65 per cent, 25-35 per cent with Stage III, and a maximum of 15 per cent in Stage IV. These figures are very broad guides, and do not take into account the circumstances particular to each individual.

Treatment of recurrent and residual disease

In some women the disease may reoccur within the first six months of treatment, possibly as a result of residual disease. In the following years there may also be recurrence of cancer in the cervical or pelvic region. The doctor may decide that if radiotherapy has failed to destroy the disease completely, the best potential outlook in patients who are capable of withstanding major surgery is **exenteration** (removal of organs within the pelvis which have been invaded by cancerous cells). This operation can involve removal of the bladder, uterus, and cervix (anterior exenteration), or the rectum, uterus, and cervix (posterior exenteration), or removal of the bladder, urethra, cervix, uterus, vagina and rectum (total exenteration). The five-year survival following exenteration is reasonable (30-60 per cent) in women with advanced but localized disease. For younger women whose sexual function is threatened by exenteration, there may be the possibility of reconstruction of the genital tract.

Chemotherapy

Chemotherapy is the treatment of illness with chemicals. Many cancers have been successfully treated with anti-cancer drugs which have been developed in the last 20 years. However, such drugs do not seem to have great effect in improving the outlook for victims of advanced cervical cancer. But now the introduction of targeting techniques which may help to direct drugs specifically to cancerous tissue, is being investigated and may one day get rid of the need for radiotherapy and surgery. However, it is more likely that this will become an adjunct to both these treatments.

Overall survival rates

Survival rates from cervical cancer are good in comparison to other forms of cancer. Much depends on the stage of cervical cancer—whether cancer cells have entered the blood stream and lodged elsewhere where they may develop into tumours which cannot be excised in the same way as they can from the cervix.

Table 9 **Cancer Survival: 1979 Registrations in England and Wales**

Age	No. patients	1 year	3 years	5 years
15-24	35	88.6	71.5	68.7
25-34	448	88.0	74.6	73.3
35-44	533	88.9	75.0	72.3
45-54	616	78.6	59.4	56.0
55-64	950	78.7	60.0	54.3
65-74	740	70.1	49.6	45.9
75-84	304	46.9	35.0	32.8
85 +	74	28.6	22.5	13.2

Source: Office of Population Censuses and Surveys.

These rates are adjusted using standard life table probabilities of surviving each period, i.e. there is a statistical likelihood of death in each age group irrespective of cervical cancer so the statistics must be adjusted to take account of this fact.

Chapter 8

Cervical cancer and contraception

- Most contraceptive methods are unlikely to cause cervical cancer.

- Combined oral contraceptives and some injectable contraceptives may act as co-factors for long-term users.

- Barrier methods of contraception exert a protective effect against cervical cancer.

- Barrier methods of contraception (condoms and vaginal or cervical caps) are preferable following local ablative treatment or cone biopsy.

Barrier contraceptives capture semen and other penile discharges and so the female genital tract is protected against infections. These infections include *Trichomonas*, gonorrhoea, syphilis, and possibly herpes. Protection is also afforded against the human papilloma virus which has been implicated in the induction of cervical cancer.

Protection is only provided as long as the condom is used for every act of intercourse and used correctly. In other words, it should be applied before any penile contact with the female genital tract. The protection fails if the condom bursts or if the infection exists in the other parts of the genital tract not covered by the condom, for example, in the vulva, vagina, thighs or scrotum. The material from which the condom is made should conform to a high manufacturing standard. In Britain, condoms should conform to BSI specifications.

The evidence supporting the protective effect of condoms has been shown in a UK study where the relative risk of severe CIN was shown to be 0.2 per 1000 woman years after 10 years of condom or diaphragm use, as compared with 4.0 per 1000 woman years for oral contraceptive use.

An American study has shown that a woman who has already had an abnormal smear is less likely to progress to severe smear abnormality if her partner uses condoms. As there was no control group in this study that is, there was no comparison with a similar group of women who continued without condoms, the study needs to be repeated by others before its conclusions are confirmed.

Condoms should be used as the choice of contraceptive method following recent local CIN treatment of the cervix, as the cervix is more susceptible to infection at this stage. In situations where a pre-cancer has occurred, the future use of a condom may protect the cervix against seminal discharges and infective organisms and a possible recurrence of the disease.

The mechanical barrier provided by vaginal diaphragm (cervical caps) protects the cervix against exposure to the contents of semen in a similar way to condoms. Nevertheless, these are released in the lower part of the genital tract and some may survive and infect the lower part of the vagina as well as the upper part and cervix.

A comparison of the incidence of CIN in barrier and non-barrier contraceptive users in the Oxford/FPA study showed the oral contraceptive users was 0.95 per 1000 woman years, for IUD users 0.85, and 0.23 for diaphragm users.

Spermicides

If spermicides are used with or without a diaphragm, they may help keep a variety of infecting organisms at bay but will not afford protection against cervical neoplasia if used alone without a diaphragm.

Combined Oral Contraceptives

Few drugs have had more stringent and rigorous testing and follow-up than oral contraceptives. Some studies have suggested that there is a link between the use of combined oral contraceptives (which contain oestrogen and progesterone) and cervical cancer. One particularly large study into the effects of the Pill involving 7000 women (Oxford University/Family Planning Association, 1983), showed that the incidence of all forms of cervical neoplasia combined was 0.9 per 1000 woman years for women on the Pill for two years, compared with 2.2 per 1000 woman years after 8 years. In the study of women using an IUD, no such increase was observed. The thirteen cases of invasive cancer which occurred were all among the combined oral contraceptive (COC) users.

A World Health Organization study (1985) showed that there was a 53 per cent increase in the risk of invasive cervical cancer among women who had taken oral contraceptives for more than five years, taking into account age of first intercourse and the number of sexual partners. The problem with this study was that it did not take into account the sexual behaviour characteristics of each woman's partner or whether they smoked.

In 1977 a study by Elizabeth Stern in California showed that the rate of progression of CIN to carcinoma *in situ* was higher in Pill users than in IUD users. It is just possible that the Pill may act as a weak co-factor. However, a study at the Margaret Pike Centre on the progression of smears showed no such effect.

In this excellent book *The Pill* (Oxford University Press, 1983), Dr John Guillebaud concluded that there was no evidence to suggest that oral contraceptives were cancer-causing agents and were more likely to act as a weak co-factor in long term users, and that their influence was many times less than the influence of sexual lifestyle.

The effects of combined oral contraceptives on the transformation zone is that in some cases the size of TZ increases rapidly (erosion), thus providing a larger area on which pre-cancerous changes may begin. Whether this actually makes women more susceptible to infection has yet to be proven.

Many centres consider that if an abnormal cervical smear has been reported, oral contraceptives can be continued as usual, even subsequent to treatment for a CIN, unless there are other reasons (unconnected with cervical CIN) for its discontinuance. However, some centres consider the oral contraceptive to be contraindicated when CIN is being treated, and prefer to recommend barrier methods of contraception.

Progesterone-only pill

There is no evidence that the progesterone-only pill causes or increases the likelihood of cervical pre-cancer. It is likely that other lifestyle aspects of women on these pills may make them more at risk of cervical cancer.

Injectable contraceptives

A World Health Organization report suggested a slightly increased risk of cervical cancer in Depo-Provera (DMPA) users, but as with oral contraceptives, the risk may not be one of direct causation and may be the result of other factors such as sexual behaviour and cigarette smoking.

IUD

There is no link between IUDs and cervical cancer.

Chapter 9

Cervical cancer and pregnancy

- Women should have a smear before contemplating pregnancy.
- Treatment before pregnancy is advisable and is extremely unlikely to have any adverse effects on fertility or a woman's capacity to carry a pregnancy to term.
- Smears during pregnancy are safe, and should be performed if missed before commencing pregnancy.
- Abnormal smears during pregnancy must be further investigated by colposcopy where possible.
- Colposcopy is safe during pregnancy and is essential to identify the abnormality and exclude the presence of an invasive cancer.
- Most abnormalities can be safely left for treatment until after pregnancy.
- If invasion is suspected, a cone biopsy may be needed. The earlier it is performed, the less likely it is that miscarriage will result.
- Pregnancy does not affect the progress of CIN, but can accelerate the progression of an invasive cancer.

With greater numbers of women under the age of 35 presenting themselves with abnormal smears, all women intending to become pregnant should have a cervical smear beforehand. The result should be known and any treatment necessary should be carried out and be successful before they start their pregnancy.

Local ablative (destructive) treatment (LAT) of cervical precancer *before* pregnancy is highly recommended, effective and in no way presents any risk to future fertility and deliveries.

Smears during pregnancy

Many women go to their doctor for the first time when they become pregnant and at that time the doctor may take the opportunity of carrying out a smear. If it is the first time a woman has had a smear this will be the first opportunity to detect an abnormality. This is especially relevant to older women at their first pregnancy who have not previously had smears. Many such women, who have deferred their first pregnancy, may have had more years of sexual activity and a greater number of partners than their younger counterparts, and are thus at greater risk of having developed a pre-cancer.

It is safe to take smears during pregnancy, but they may sometimes be reported as showing no endocervical cells because of changes in the cervix at this time and also there is a reluctance by the sampler to collect cells from the endocervical canal of a pregnant woman. Such smears may therefore be regarded as incomplete and may have to be repeated after the delivery.

It is not an ideal situation to smear during pregnancy—one would prefer the woman to have had a smear and treatment of any abnormality beforehand. The finding of an abnormality during pregnancy will cause anxiety in the mother-to-be as well as potential problems if the abnormality is too severe to be left untreated.

It is important to have a smear taken during pregnancy if this test has not been recently performed. The vast majority of smears taken during pregnancy are normal but about 15-20 abnormal smears are reported per thousand pregnancies.

Abnormal smears

Those pregnant women whose smear is reported as abnormal need to have a repeat smear and further investigation by colposcopy. Colposcopy during pregnancy is a completely safe, pain-less and important investigation which in no way harms the mother or the baby. However, during pregnancy, colposcopy needs to be performed by a very experienced colposcopist because a pregnant cervix has a very different appearance than a non-pregnant cervix and it may be difficult to interpret what the col-poscopy reveals.

Most colposcopic examinations which follow an abnormal smear reveal minor areas of abnormalities. As long as the entire abnormal area is easily visible and the overall impression is that of a localized and early CIN, the experienced colposcopist may be able to observe the disturbance, leaving it unbiopsied and untreated until after the delivery. If CIN is discovered during pregnancy, at least one further colposcopic observation should be performed, although more may be needed according to individual circumstances and availability of colposcopic facilities.

Pregnancy does not accelerate the progression of the CIN, and as most CINs take many years to progress into more severe stages, the mother can be allowed to continue her pregnancy without any fear of invasive disease if the state of the cervix is carefully monitored. Furthermore, the pre-cancer is unlikely to affect the baby in any way.

Six weeks after the delivery, a further colposcopic examina-tion with an accompanying smear and biopsy should be per-formed and, if the abnormality persists, treatment will be recommended. Occasionally it is found that the abnormality has disappeared completely, but a further smear should be taken six months later, and if it is clear, then another one should be taken a year later.

Biopsies in pregnancy

Taking a biopsy in pregnancy is a very rare event and usually only performed if invasive cancer is suspected. When indicated, a wedge biopsy, a special kind of biopsy which involves a very thin wedge of tissue for histological examination, is taken. The problem with taking any biopsy is that the pregnant cervix has a lot of blood vessels in it, so even small biopsies may cause a lot of bleeding. Occasionally, a colposcopic biopsy may be taken during the early stages of pregnancy where neither the patient nor colposcopist are aware of the pregnancy. This will not cause a miscarriage, but doctors generally avoid taking biopsies in pregnancy.

Local treatment in pregnancy

If the colposcopy, with or without biopsy, shows the presence of localized CIN, it is safer and preferable to wait until after the pregnancy to have local treatment because there is a small risk of inducing an abortion or premature delivery as a result of such treatment.

Cone biopsy

Before the advent of colposcopy, when the cervix appeared normal to the naked eye although the smear was persistently abnormal, cone biopsy was usually carried out.

During pregnancy this procedure was complicated by abortion, premature labour, cervical scarring and worst of all by haemorrhage, frequently necessitating blood transfusion, and occasionally hysterectomy, and sometimes resulting in death. Such complications occurred in a quarter to a third of all patients. For these reasons, the obstetrician therefore tended to limit the cone biopsy. As a result, cone biopsies carried out during pregnancy, especially during the second and third trimester, when a severe grade of CIN was present, failed to completely cut out the diseased tissue in 40 per cent of cases. Many obstetricians were tempted simply to postpone investigations of an abnormal smear until after birth, so that occasionally an invasive but hidden carcinoma had been allowed to grow.

In recent years, most, if not all, British gynaecology departments have been equipped with a colposcope, and pregnant women now have a much better chance than they used to of being seen by an experienced colposcopist. The colposcopist should be able to distinguish between an early CIN, which may be left until the end of pregnancy before treatment, and an invasive cancer, which would need immediate treatment if the woman is to have the maximum chance of long-term survival.

As cone biopsy can now be carefully directed under colposcopic surveillance, the procedure is now far safer and more accurate, increasing the likelihood of removing all the diseased tissue during conization. The operative complications previously associated with cone biopsy have also been greatly reduced. If a cone biopsy needs to be performed during the first three months of pregnancy then the risk of losing the baby is very small. This treatment carries a much greater risk from four to five months pregnant (mid-trimester) onwards. As with many cone biopsies, hospital admission, and a general anaesthetic are required. A cone-shaped piece of cervical tissue is removed and this may weaken the cervix which will subsequently not be able to maintain the hold that the cervix has on the pregnant uterus. A stitch can be inserted around the cervix to reinforce its hold on the pregnancy.

Depending on the results of the cone biopsy, if the removal of the disease has been complete and there is no invasion, then a vaginal delivery is attempted and the Shirodkar stitch is removed just before the delivery. However, if the disease is more advanced, for instance a microinvasion (up to three millimetres beneath the basement membrane), then a vaginal delivery is not advised for fear of spreading the disease into the lymphatic and blood channels as a result of the physical pressures on the cervical tissues arising from the birth. In these circumstances, the baby should be delivered by Caesarean section.

Invasive cancer during pregnancy

Although pregnancy does not accelerate the progression of CIN, it can speed up the progress of invasive cancer to more severe forms. This highlights the need for smears to be taken before the onset of pregnancy, and treatment to be performed if an invasion is detected.

Treating invasive cancer

In Stages Ib and IIa, where the cancer is confined to the womb or the womb and the top of the vagina, it is necessary to perform a radical abdominal hysterectomy, including removal of the Fallopian tubes (with conservation of both ovaries if possible) the removal of pelvic lymph nodes, and a 3-4 cm 'cuff' from the top of the vagina where it attaches to the uterus. If this operation is carried out in the first or second trimester the uterus is removed with the baby inside it. At this stage, it is too early for the baby to survive.

When the disease is identified at six months pregnancy, it is possible to save the baby by giving the mother corticosteroids which help to ripen the baby's lungs which are always at risk during premature delivery. The baby is then delivered by Caesarean section and a radical hysterectomy is performed as described above.

In more advanced cancer (IIb and beyond) where surgery is of limited value, radiotherapy has to be given. If this happens in the early stages of pregnancy, there may be spontaneous abortion of the foetus. However, if this condition is discovered in the third trimester, then a Caesarean section is performed before radiotherapy is begun, thereby saving the baby. In cases of invasive cervical cancer, decisions on treatment should be reched by joint consultation of the patient with the gynaecologist, radiotherapist, pathologist and neonatologist (doctors specializing in the care of premature babies).

Chapter 10

Cervical cancer and post-menopausal women

- Post-menopausal women need regular cervical smears, at least once every three years.

- Smears should be performed annually on women who have had pre-cancerous or cancerous conditions in the genital region including women who have had a hysterectomy for such conditions.

- Although a woman may have ceased having sex, her or her partner's previous sexual activities may have resulted in a pre-cancerous change which may not manifest itself until many years later.

- Virginal women or those with little history of sexual intercourse, should still have smears as these may detect pelvic cancers not associated with sexual intercourse.

- Any bleeding or vaginal discharge after menopause is an indication for immediate investigation which should include a pelvic examination and cervical smear at the very least.

- Post-menopausal women are at greatest risk from cervical cancer, mainly because they do not present themselves for screening.

Post-menopausal women have traditionally regarded themselves as being immune to cervical cancer. Consequently, they are the least likely group of women to present themselves for screening.

They are most likely to present when signs and symptoms such as bleeding or pelvic pain cause them to seek medical attention by which time the disease, if present, may be very advanced, major surgery may be required and it may be too late to save the patient's life.

Post-menopausal women do not attend family planning or antenatal clinics and may have no need to visit their medical practitioner for any other reason. Unless they receive and respond to a specific request to present themselves for a smear, they are not likely to remember and initiate such an appointment. Some women, despite receiving a recall appointment for the cervical smear test, ignore it and fail to turn up. This may be because of the (mistaken) belief that they are unlikely to be at risk of this disease.

The history of a post-menopausal woman's sexual partners may also have a bearing on her likelihood of having cervical cancer. Such history may often not be known to them. A cervical pre-cancer which began many years previously may only now be progressing to a more serious abnormality. Another risk factor is one of age itself as immunity gradually lowers, consequently increasing susceptibility to cancerous changes. Such changes may have been lurking undetected for many years if a woman has not had regular cervical smears.

How can such women be reached? Publicity and information regarding the need to attend for smears may reach them via their medical practitioners in the shape of a recall appointment, but often such an invitation does little to inform them how they should relate to the need for such a test. In the absence of recall, their daughters, husbands, or informed friends who may have attended for such tests, should encourage them to go. Occasionally other female members of the family may have had or known someone who has had the disease, and they should take it upon themselves to encourage other women to have smears.

Articles in the press and programmes on TV may alert some of the older women and it is hoped that the current generation of post-menopausal women will utilize such information and respond to the need for having a regular cervical smear.

The disease which appears in post-menopausal women is

difficult to detect because it is very often hidden deep and high inside the endocervical canal. This is sometimes caused by the post-menopausal changes which pull the squamocolumnar junction and transformation zone up into the endocervical canal, and sometimes by operative procedures on the cervices of these women. This poses the problem of inadequate sampling of these cells and falsely negative results. By having a regular smear, every three years or less, the chances of detecting the disease are increased. It must be emphasized that 60-90 per cent of women who die from cervical cancer either have not had a smear at all or have had one more than five years ago.

The sampling technique involves the use of a special spatula able to enter the cervical canal. Ideally, the person taking the sample should be trained to appreciate the problems in sampling the endocervical canal of a post-menopausal woman. A technique for improving the chances of taking an adequate smear is the 'oestrogen test'. This involves daily pre-treatment with 10 microgrammes of oestrogen for ten days which reduces tightening of the endocervical canal and will allow access to, and easier sampling of, this area. If colposcopy is needed, such pre-treatment will also allow for good examination. There is no 'withdrawal bleeding' associated with the end of hormonal treatment.

The changing hormonal pattern in post-menopausal women, especially the decreased levels of ovarian hormones, may make the cervical and endocervical cells appear shrivelled and thin (atrophic) and inflammatory changes may be reported. These changes may either hide a cervical carcinoma or be a sign of one. Hormone replacement therapy may also produce changes in the cells, so the cytological picture has to be viewed in conjunction with the patient's case history and particular attention paid to results of previous cervical smears and sexual and obstetric history. In some of these women, where the oestrogen has little effect or had not been given, colposcopy may be unsatisfactory because the stenosed canal cannot properly be inspected, and a cone biopsy may be necessary. Pelvic examination and smears are essential if there is any bleeding, however slight. The same applies if there is any unusual vaginal discharge or abdominal, pelvic, rectal or bladder discomfort.

Smears after hysterectomy

Many women are unaware that they should continue to have regular smears even after they have had a hysterectomy and so they may not see themselves at risk. However, although the cervix may have been removed during hysterectomy, it is still possible for pre-cancer or cancer to begin in the remaining vaginal skin deep in the vaginal vault where it was once attached to the cervix. It is also possible for the vagina itself to develop pre-cancer (called VAIN—vaginal intraepithelial neoplasia) or cancer in the side walls or on the vulva which will be detected by the smear. Women who have had a hysterectomy for non-cancerous reasons, should continue to have a smear at least once every three years. Pelvic examination at that time screens for ovarian and pelvic masses.

Women who have had a hysterectomy as a result of a pre-cancer or cancer will need to have a follow-up arranged by their consultant. This should include colposcopy and a smear and, if there is no sign of recurrent malignancy after two years, then annual smears should be continued. Post-menopausal women who are still virgins or have rarely had sexual intercourse, and are under 70, should still have smears until they have had three consecutive negative results prior to their 70th birthday. These may pick up cancers which are not thought to be associated with sexual intercourse such as adenocarcinoma of the cervical canal or a cancer in the body of the uterus whose cells may pass down the canal and be picked up by the smear. (Adenocarcinoma occurs most often in women between 60 and 70.)

Hormone replacement therapy

As far as is known, there is no evidence to show that HRT triggers off any pre-cancerous or cancerous changes in the cervix. Past history of cervical pre-cancer or cancer is not *per se* a contraindication to hormone replacement therapy. Provided that there are no other contraindications, such as breast cancer, hypertension, kidney, gall bladder disease or increased blood clotting, the hormone replacement therapy may be given under regular medical supervision to replace the naturally diminishing ovarian hormonal production.

Combined oestrogen/progesterone preparations are given to those women who have not had a hysterectomy. Oestrogen (single) hormone preparation may be given to women who have had their uterus removed.

Hormone replacement therapy should relieve hot flushes, protect against bone loss (osteoporosis), prevent ageing changes in the urethra and vagina, and protect against cardiovascular disease.

Chapter 11

The role of men in cervical cancer

- Men play an important role in the spread of cervical cancer.
- Genital warts caused by the human papilloma virus have been implicated as potential agents of induction.
- Genital warts are not always visible, but can sometimes be detected under microscopic observation using a colposcope.
- Barrier methods of contraception, such as condoms, can protect women from potential pre-cancer-inducing agents present in semen.
- Men whose partners develop cervical cancer rarely develop penile cancer. However, the evidence of the presence of wart virus is found in 35-40 per cent of penile cancers.
- Women whose male partners have penile cancers are at increased risk of developing cervical cancer.
- Curtailing the number of sexual partners, stopping smoking (both partners), encouraging smear tests in women partners, checking for genital warts in both partners, and the use of condoms can diminish the risk of a woman developing a cervical cancer.

From everything that has been written in this book so far, it is clear that there is a link between sexual intercourse and cervical cancer. As this book is primarily aimed at women, the information has been biased towards them. However, if cervical cancer is a consequence of sexual intercourse, then **men** obviously share some of the responsibility.

Most men would probably not think of cancer as a sexually transmitted disease in the way that they might consider syphilis or gonorrhoea. After all, cancer isn't contagious, or is it? The fact remains that a lot of evidence has pointed towards some men being carriers of agents which induces cervical cancer in their sexual partners.

There is some evidence that the impact of semen on the cervix alters the surface characteristics of the cervical skin which may progress to pre-cancer. One particular substance identified as the cause is 'basic protein', proteins found in large quantities on the surface of sperm, which causes potentially damaging changes to the cells' genetic material, although how is not yet known. In a joint study between a team of doctors in Sydney and Albert Singer, a gynaecological consultant in Sheffield (who is now at the Whittington and Royal Northern Hospitals in London), it was shown that there was a significant difference in the basic protein content of semen from men in different social classes (Read, B.L. *et al*, *Lancet*, 1978 volume 2, p. 60). Men in social class I (upper and upper middle), whose wives are at the least risk of cervical cancer, were shown to have a small amount of basic protein in their semen in comparison to the high amount detected in men from social class V (lower working), whose wives have a relatively high risk of contracting the disease.

Another agent implicated in cervical cancer is the human papilloma virus (HPV) which was first identified as a possible cause of CIN in the late 1970s. Several studies have since supported this observation. For example, one study showed that, in a group of women who had CIN 3 or carcinoma *in situ* and whose partners were carriers of the HPV, 95 per cent of the women had the same type of wart virus in their cancer cells as in the genital tracts of the men.

Some men will know that they are carriers of HPV because the penile skin may react to the presence of the virus to form a wart — hence the common name of 'wart virus'. They look similar to warts found on skin elsewhere on the body, such as on the hands, but tend to stand out a little more. They may be treated by the local application of a paint such as podophyllin which burns the wart off. This is usually done in hospital but can be self-administered. However, as there may be a lot of pain, it is advisable to have the treatment in hospital so that the treatment dose is carefully applied and controlled. Where the facilities exist, laser treatment is faster and more effective in removing warts. It is not known how effective this method is in attacking and eradicating the virus from the genital tract, but it has been suggested that the treatment may induce an immune response which helps to overcome the infection.

Many men are unaware that they are carriers of the virus because the warts may be so small that the only way of detecting them is by colposcopy. In some cases, the virus may be present without any signs at all although the presence of HPV can be demonstrated by special staining techniques.

As the wart virus can be transferred from women to uninfected men, the more partners a man has, the more likely he is to become infected and spread the infection to others. The virus is likely to remain a permanent fixture in the genital tract, and it can be spread very easily. The only clue that a man has that he has been infected is the presence of warts or knowledge of his partner's warts.

Men are perhaps not so concerned about being infected with the virus as women because they are not affected by it except for the unsightly presence of warts. However, the fact that they may be transmitting the virus to previously uninfected women who may suffer a cervical pre-cancer or cancer as a result, should be taken into consideration.

While men can be put into high risk (of inducing cervical cancer) groups by their sexual behaviour and social class, the second broad category into which they can be classified is by occupation as indicated in table 10 (see also table 5 in chapter 2).

The differences in occupational groups are thought to be due to their working conditions, where they may be exposed to certain chemicals which appear in traces on the genital region or in the semen. The partners of men who smoke have been shown to be at increased risk of cervical cancer. It may be that different occupational groups have different sexual behaviour patterns.

What can men do to prevent themselves inducing cervical cancer in their partners? Men should bear in mind their own sexual and smoking history and whether any of their previous partners developed cervical cancer. This could give them an indication that they may be potentially high-risk partners and should thus consider barrier contraception such as a condom. A further sign that a man should consider using a condom is the presence of genital warts or discharge which can indicate the presence of HPV. As mentioned, warts can be treated to some extent, although this may fail to eradicate the virus from the genital tract. Again, if a man belongs to a high risk group by occupation, he can also protect his partner by using a condom.

Table 10 **Standardized mortality ratios above 120 of husbands in England and Wales (1970-72) of wives aged 15-64 with cervical cancer**

Occupation	Standardized mortality ratio
Armed forces	201
Miners and quarrymen	185
Labourers not elsewhere classified	174
Furnacemen, forge, foundry, rolling mill workers	170
Glass and ceramics makers	163
Gas, coke and chemical makers	160
Food, drink and tobacco workers	151
Painters and decorators	147
Construction workers	146
Leather workers	143
Transport and communication workers	138
Service, sport and recreation workers	134
Drivers of stationary engines and cranes	121

Source: Occupational mortality. Registrar General's Decennial Supplement for England and Wales 1970-72.

The use of condoms should only be discounted if the relationship is monogamous (neither partner is having sexual intercourse with other partners) and the man has not slept with any women who have subsequently developed cervical cancer. Good genital hygiene, which should include washing before and after sexual intercourse, is also important. But perhaps the most helpful thing that men can do is to ensure that their partner has a regular cervical smear.

A question men often ask is, 'Why has my partner developed cervical cancer while I have not developed cancer of the penis?' The answer may lie in the fact that the skin and mucus lining of the penis is made up of different types of cells from those found on the surface of the cervix and the cervical skin seems to form a particularly hospitable site for infection and cancerous change. It may also be because of the difference between the male and female hormonal systems. It is worth saying that, in the small number of men who do develop penile cancer, their sexual partners are prone to developing cervical cancer, and presence of the HPV is found in 35-40 per cent of penile cancers.

Chapter 12

Psychological problems

- Fear, anxiety and depression are among the emotions felt by many women faced with the news that they have a cervical abnormality.

- Breakdown of sexual relationships may be a consequence of the discovery of cervical cancer or pre-cancer.

- Women and their partners need careful explanation and counselling and careful follow-up after treatment.

- Inadequate explanations or prolonged waiting for treatment, will add to fear and anxiety.

- Many women may experience some loss of libido due to fear and worry about the disease.

Anxiety and fear

The suspicion of any abnormality in a woman's cervix raises its own problems and anxieties. There is a definite fear involved in learning that there is or might be a possibility of a cancer in an organ as 'intimate' as the cervix. Fear that one's future sexual life will in some way be impaired or destroyed; fear of having intercourse as it may cause the disease again; fear of impaired fertility and not being able to have more children as a consequence of the disease and possibly as a result of treatment; fear of not knowing what investigations and treatments will take place;

fear of death. No matter how carefully it is explained that the abnormality may not be cancerous, or that if it is, it can be completely cured, the fear of cancer remains. The long queues and great delays for colposcopy, impose an almost unbearable mental strain on all those women who have been found to have an abnormal smear and who await further tests. As one woman put it recently, 'During those six months of waiting and not knowing what was going to be found, I felt like throwing myself under a bus.' Even if a smear is reported as being indicative of a pre-cancer, the only word a frightened woman seems to hear is 'cancer'. Despite reassurances that statistics show the local treatment of CIN to be safe and successful, fears and anxieties still remain after treatment, not least because of the complex explanations and need for continued testing.

With a suspect infection which may be caused by HPV, one has to explain that there is no known drug which will get rid of the wart virus entirely, and that removal of a genital wart does not remove the virus present in the genital tract of a man or a woman. This may not reassure a woman or her partner, and fear may still remain regarding recurrence of the disease. However, treatment aims to destroy the entire transformation zone and thus remove the area on the cervix which is liable to become cancerous. The new lining that regrows is of a different kind from the original transformation zone and may be less likely to become cancerous. In destroying the transformation zone it is still possible that some small areas which harbour abnormal cells have failed to be eradicated and it is possible for the disease either to reoccur or for a new disease to develop. This is why regular follow-ups are needed to detect any further occurrence of abnormality.

The necessity of follow-ups creates further fear of recurrence of the disease, especially because follow-up suggests an expectation that the disease may occur again. A woman may also ask, 'What is the point of just curing me? I go home and I will be infected by my partner again. Why isn't he being examined and treated?' The anxieties do not just affect women. Men often ask, 'What can I do, how can I be examined and how can you treat me and cure me so that my partner does not get infected again?'

Following treatment, or even while awaiting it, some women experience a loss of sex drive. The knowledge that one's partner may have been instrumental in transmitting this disease may cause a whole range of psychosexual difficulties. As there is such an enormous number of possible causes to suspect, it is impossible to be very specific in advising partners what exactly they should do to prevent the disease other than keeping to monogamous relationships and being aware of the risk factors that have already been described, and making use of the cervical cytology screening services that are available.

There is no way to eradicate all the factors which may be responsible for transmitting this disease but we can alter our approach and understanding of what should be happening. It may take a generation before people understand that women *need* this kind of screening and that they will need this kind of caution in order to protect themselves from dying unnecessarily. It is also very difficult for patients (and sometimes their doctors) to understand why the laboratory keeps asking for repeat smears again and again.

Embarrassment

There is embarrassment and consequent reluctance towards being examined in what is, after all, a very vulnerable position, in which the very intimate and hidden personal recesses of a woman's genital area are being explored. The fact that the examination may be in the presence of male staff, staff who may be known socially to a patient, or other personnel who are there for training purposes may also contribute to apprehension and worry. However, one must weigh up the fact that one's life may well be at risk and that doctors make intimate examinations of thousands of women every year.

Guilt

Some women feel guilty that they may have cervical cancer because the disease has been associated with promiscuous behaviour, although, as we have shown, this does not reflect the true situation. They may blame themselves for having an affair which brought them disease. However, one incidence of sexual intercourse may be enough to induce the onset of cervical cancer.

Suspicion

Frequently, when a woman is faithful to one man, the discovery that she has cervical cancer can lead to suspicion that her partner has been involved in sexual relations with another woman. However, the initiation of pre-cancer or cancer may have taken place a long time before it was diagnosed, and the onset of disease can be a reflection of events that occurred before a relationship started. Furthermore, cervical cancer can occur in women where both she and her partner have only ever made love to each other. In this case, the cervical cancer may be in the form of adenocarcinoma which is not thought to be sexually transmissible.

Anger

Anger may be directed in lots of ways, many of which may be unexpressed. A woman may be angry at the unfairness that she is one of the unlucky ones and the thought that her disease may have been acquired as a result of her partner's infidelity. There may also be anger at doctors or other medical staff because they have diagnosed cancer and the patient is not able to understand what the diagnosis means. In areas where there is a lack of facilities, there may be anger at long delays in evaluating smears and at having no written explanation on the progression of the disease, its treatment and prognosis, and anger at not being able to have a complete cure once and for all.

There is a great need for medical staff to take time and show tact, gentleness and understanding when dealing with stressed and often frightened women. Under stress, such women may not always understand what is being said to them. Unfortunately, with the enormous pressure of work, medical staff often do not have enough time to spend with each patient.

Women who have suffered psychological problems as described above, can get information, advice and counselling from centres listed at the end of this book.

Chapter 13

Control of cervical cancer — the worldwide position

- The cervical cancer death rate has fallen in countries which have introduced a comprehensive cervical screening programme.

- In both developed and developing nations the incidence of the disease increases up to the age of 35, then the incidence remains about the same until around 60, after which it declines.

- The incidence (number of positive cases per smears taken) of pre-cancer has increased substantially over the last decade.

Screening

The aim of screening is to identify the disease before it becomes cancerous and thus reduce the incidence of fully developed cervical cancer and the subsequent death from it. In the developed world, screening has been going on for some thirty years.

Well-organized screening programmes have been very effective. In the Nordic countries, which introduced screening in the mid-sixties, Denmark, Iceland, Sweden and Finland have all shown a decrease in incidence of ill health and mortality from the disease. In fact, Iceland showed a 60 per cent reduction in mortality over a 10-year period. In Canada, screening resulted in the incidence of cervical cancer falling from 29.4 to 6.9 per

100,000 women, and mortality from 11.4 to 3.3 per 100,000 women during a 20-year screening programme in British Columbia.

In countries such as the Nordic nations, Canada and the USA, some 60 per cent of the population are covered by screening at regular intervals. However, in many developing nations screening is non-existent or sporadic.

Here are a few examples, provided by the World Health Organization (from: *Bulletin of the World Health Organization* 1986, volume 64(4), p.607), of different programmes which exist around the world.

India Cytological screening is restricted to large urban centres which also have facilities for diagnosis and treatment. It is estimated that even if there were a twelve-fold increase in trained staff by the year 2000, only 25 per cent of all women in India would be screened.

Indonesia Screening tends to be linked to family planning programmes and is available in only a few hospitals. More than 55 per cent of women screened are under 30 years of age although only 7 per cent of cervical cancer patients occur in that group.

Chile This country has 16 cytological laboratories which recruit women mostly through maternal and child health/family planning programmes. There is capacity for screening 500,000 smears a year which could theoretically cater for all women between 35 and 60 (around two million) to be screened every five years.

Hungary Cytology screening began in 1972 and is performed in 72 laboratories throughout the country which have the capability to screen all women between the age of 20 and 65 every three years.

China Screening began as long ago as 1957 in Beijing, later being extended to other large cities. Some districts have annual, biannual or triannual screenings. During the last 15 years, 16 million women have been screened, a small proportion of the nation's total, but understandable when one considers how large and widespread the population is.

The World Health Organization recently stated that approximately 50 per cent of adult women in developed countries, and less than 5 per cent in developing countries have been screened in the last five years. Developed countries tend to concentrate their screening on younger women under 35.

Cost-effective screening intervals

Studies of screening programmes in eight European countries and North America show that for women in the 35-64 age range, the reduction in incidence of invasive cancer from screening every two years is as great as that from annual screening, and that the reduction from screening every three years is nearly as great. Even screening every 10 years gives a 64 per cent reduction in risk. Screening all women every ten years is more effective than screening 50 per cent of women every five years. Overall, age is the most important risk factor in considering the design of screening programmes.

Although there has been a considerable increase in the number of young women under 35 who have contracted cervical pre-cancer, the invasive disease is rare in women under 25. In both developed and developing countries, the incidence of invasive cervical cancer increases up to the age of 35 after which the incidence remains about the same until around 60 and then declines.

Effectiveness of screening

Despite widespread early detection screening programmes in developed countries, more than 60 per cent of patients are initially diagnosed with evidence of considerable local spread and metastases of the cancer cells into lymph nodes in the pelvis or other parts of the body. The International Federation of Gynaecology and Obstetrics analysed information from 32,000 patients with cervical cancer from 120 cancer centres in developed countries and found that cancer was spread as shown in Table 10.

The figures in Table 11 clearly show the benefits of early detection in terms of long-term survival, particularly as long-term survival among properly diagnosed and treated CIN patients is almost 100 per cent.

Table 11

Stage	Five year survival rate
I — 33%	78%
II — 36%	57%
III — 27%	31%
IV — 4%	8%

Source: Petterson, F. *et al.*, 1985. ed. *Annual report on the results of treatment in gynaecological cancer*. Stockholm, International Federation of Gynaecology and Obstetrics.

As financial constraints prevent many countries implementing effective screening programmes, the World Health Organization recommends that the aim should be to screen all women between the ages of 35 and 40 at least once in their lifetime and if more resources become available, the frequency of screening should be increased to once every five or ten years between the ages of 35 to 55. The WHO ideal is one in which all women between the ages of 25 and 60 are screened once every three years.

Screening in Great Britain

Table 12 Cervical cancer: deaths and screening

Great Britain	Thousands and percentages							
	1976	1981	1982	1983	1984	1985	1986	1987[1]
Deaths	2.4	2.2	2.1	2.2	2.1	2.2	2.2	2.1
Smears taken	2,923	3,442	3,378	3,669	3,911	4,455	4,468	4,754
Smears as a percentage of women aged 15 and over	13.3	15.2	14.8	16.0	17.0	19.3	19.2	20.4

[1] 1987 figures for England relate to the financial year ending 31 March 1988.

Source: Department of Health, Scottish Health Service Common Services Agency, Welsh Office.

In Great Britain, the number of smears taken has increased annually from 7,000 in 1965, to 2.9 million in 1976, and to 4.7 million in the year ending March 1988. The number of women eligible for smears is around 17.5 million.

Table 12 shows that nationally, the death rate has been reduced to just over 200 women per annum. Critics of high intensity screening would argue that little change in the death rate has been achieved, despite a massive increase in screening. However, this must be balanced against the fact that there are a far larger number of positive smears being detected (see tables 14 and 15).

Table 13 **Cervical cytology: Positive results and deaths detected in England and Wales**

	Number of positive results			Number of deaths from cervical cancer		
	1981	1986	1987-88[4]	1981	1986	1987
Northern	6.8	11.0	11.7	89.3	91.8	84.9
Yorkshire	7.8	8.8	8.3	94.6	81.1	85.9
Trent	4.7	6.8	9.2	87.5	86.6	71.2
East Anglia	8.5	12.4	12.8	72.7	68.0	65.3
North West Thames	6.2	7.6	9.7	50.9	71.1	49.3
North East Thames	7.1	9.3	9.7	62.2	72.8	53.6
South East Thames	5.9	7.4	9.9	76.5	80.4	71.1
South West Thames	5.3	7.1	7.6	63.9	49.5	59.4
Wessex	8.1	6.7	5.8	62.8	57.0	65.8
Oxford	6.4	7.2	7.9	51.8	57.0	60.3
South Western	8.6	12.3	11.4	75.5	73.7	88.1
West Midlands	7.1	10.1	8.3	76.0	66.3	74.8
Mersey	9.1	13.6	13.1	115.8	105.2	99.8
North Western	9.2	13.5	15.6	103.8	104.3	86.3
England	7.0	9.5	10.1	78.1	76.7	72.6
Wales	8.4	8.6	8.3	91.8	95.7	90.5

Note: The number of positive results is per thousand smears examined, and the number of deaths is per one million women. 1987/88 data collected on a financial year basis for England and on a calendar year for Wales.

Source: Department of Health.

Table 12 also shows that more than a fifth of women over 15 were screened in the year ending March 1988, compared to less than a seventh of the population in 1976.

Table 13 shows how the number of positive smears (minimum CIN 3) per thousand patients has substantially increased in each region in England and Wales, almost doubling in some regions (except for Wessex) between 1981 and 1986. However, in some regions the postive rate increased only slightly, or actually decreased, between 1986 and the year ending March 1988.

The different results in each region may reflect different screening policies as well as differing social conditions, with subsequent variation in predisposing factors to cervical cancer. For example, people in the more affluent London region had among the lowest death rates.

Table 14 **Smears taken, positive results and positive results per 1,000 smears examined, 1977-1987/8 (England and Wales)**

Year	All smears (thousands)		Positive results		Positive results per 1,000 smears examined	
	No.	Index (1977 = 100)	No.	Index (1977 = 100)	No.	Index (1977 = 100)
1977	2,545	100	14,952	100	5.9	100
1978	2,587	102	16,260	109	6.3	107
1979	2,749	108	17,333	116	6.3	107
1980	2,928	115	19,923	133	6.8	115
1981	2,999	118	21,340	143	7.1	120
1982	2,951	116	22,370	150	7.6	129
1983	3,200	126	24,836	166	7.8	132
1984	3,417	134	30,331	203	8.9	151
1985	3,897	153	35,752	239	9.2	156
1986	3,908	154	37,095	248	9.5	161
1987/88	4,322	170	43,052	288	10.0	169

Source: DH Statistics & Management Information.

The number of smears taken in England and Wales has increased by 11 per cent since 1986 and 70 per cent since 1977. The number of positive results has increased by 16 per cent since

1986 and 188 per cent since 1977. Around 1 per cent of the total smear tests performed in 1987/88 were positive (CIN 3 or worse).

Table 14 also shows that the number of positive smears taken per thousand smears nearly doubled from 5.9 in 1977 to 10.0 in 1987/88.

Whether the increase in the rate, rather than the total number of positive smears, reflects better detection techniques, or an epidemic of a sexually transmitted agent such as the wart virus, or changing lifestyles such as number of partners, diet, clothing, smoking or some as yet unidentified environmental factor, is currently under debate in the medical profession.

Table 15 **Positive smears by age, 1977-1987/88 (England and Wales)**

Year	All ages	Age Under 25	25-29	30-34	35 +
1977	14,952	1,517	2,740	2,997	7,698
1978	16,260	1,708	3,216	3,554	7,777
1979	17,333	1,645	3,385	3,934	8,369
1980	19,923	2,117	4,027	4,597	9,182
1981	21,340	2,098	4,470	5,068	9,704
1982	22,370	2,382	4,729	5,151	10,108
1983	24,836	2,477	5,155	5,703	11,501
1984	30,331	3,163	6,405	6,739	14,024
1985	35,752	4,070	7,341	8,013	16,328
1986	37,095	4,625	7,521	8,002	16,947
1987/88	43,052	6,194	8,949	8,766	19,143

Source: DH Statistics & Management Information (SM12B).

Table 15 shows that since 1977 the greatest increase in positive smears occurred in the younger age groups. In the under-25 group, there has been a 308 per cent increase from 1977 to 1987/88. This may reflect an increase in the number of smears being taken from women in younger age groups.

Table 16 shows that in 1987/88, 92 per cent of positive biopsies following positive smear tests resulted in a diagnosis of dysplasia or carcinoma *in situ*, compared to 75 per cent in 1977. It also shows that the proportion of positive biopsy results leading to a diagnosis of micro-carcinoma (microinvasive carcinoma),

Table 16 **Smears detected as positive for the first time — distribution by result of biopsy, 1977-1987/88 (England and Wales)**

Year	Negative	Dysplasia	Carcinoma-in-situ	Micro-carcinoma	Invasive squamous carcinoma	Other malignant disease	Case under pre-biopsy observation	Biopsy not done or result not known
1977	4.3	16.5	38.1	3.6	10.7	3.5	9.3	13.8
1978	3.0	17.5	40.2	2.3	8.6	2.9	9.7	15.8
1979	3.6	17.3	37.5	3.0	8.1	3.3	12.7	14.5
1980	3.2	16.2	39.2	3.0	8.4	2.5	10.9	16.6
1981	2.9	21.5	40.0	3.0	7.2	1.9	8.5	15.1
1982	2.9	21.1	42.0	2.9	6.9	1.7	6.1	16.5
1983	3.8	21.7	43.6	2.8	6.4	1.9	5.2	14.6
1984	3.8	21.8	45.3	2.7	6.0	2.0	6.2	12.2

Year	Negative	CIN I mild dysplasia	CIN II moderate dysplasia	CIN III severe dysplasia and carcinoma-in-situ	Micro-carcinoma	Invasive squamous carcinoma	Other malignant disease	Case under pre-biopsy observation	Biopsy not done or result not known
1985[1]	4.7	4.1	11.2	51.7	2.9	6.3	1.5	5.2	12.5
1986[1]	3.9	4.4	12.7	52.8	2.8	5.2	1.2	4.5	12.5
1987/88[1]	5.3	6.3	12.3	50.1	1.7	3.9	0.8	5.1	14.6

[1] In 1985 the categories describing biopsy results were expanded.

Source: DH Statistics & Management Information.

143

Table 17 Deaths from cervical cancer (England and Wales)

Deaths per million in parentheses

Year	Age										All ages
	20-24	25-29	30-34	35-39	40-44	45-49	50-54	55-59	50-74	75 +	
1977	2(1)	18(10)	53(31)	74(53)	92(68)	126(89)	270(180)	262(175)	826(205)	422(234)	2145(107)
1978	1(1)	34(20)	59(33)	81(57)	82(60)	125(89)	233(159)	306(196)	803(203)	429(232)	2153(107)
1979	6(3)	27(16)	56(31)	79(54)	88(63)	137(99)	177(123)	300(186)	792(203)	425(225)	2087(103)
1980	10(6)	30(18)	74(41)	82(55)	79(57)	116(85)	189(133)	278(210)	796(201)	414(214)	2068(101)
1981	7(4)	30(18)	81(44)	89(56)	105(75)	103(76)	167(118)	251(169)	782(197)	402(203)	2017(98)
1982	7(4)	25(15)	77(44)	89(52)	113(81)	125(92)	132(94)	197(136)	784(197)	382(189)	1932(94)
1983	3(2)	43(25)	78(46)	92(52)	104(73)	127(93)	155(112)	184(130)	717(181)	456(220)	1959(95)
1984	4(2)	48(28)	59(35)	98(54)	116(79)	97(70)	144(106)	187(134)	749(190)	397(187)	1899(91)
1985	5(2)	35(20)	74(45)	134(73)	92(61)	117(84)	138(103)	185(133)	747(190)	430(199)	1957(93)
1986	3(1)	48(26)	77(46)	128(69)	138(88)	150(109)	144(108)	178(130)	724(185)	413(188)	2004(95)
1987	8(4)	43(23)	77(46)	131(74)	125(73)	124(90)	137(103)	153(112)	706(182)	399(178)	1903(90)

Source: Office of Population Censuses and Surveys.

invasive squamous carcinoma or other malignant disease fell from 25 per cent in 1977 to 8 per cent in 1987/88. This may be an encouraging sign of potential malignancies being identified earlier. However the proportion of first time positive smear tests which were shown to be negative on biopsy was 5.3 per cent, the highest rate over the last ten years.

Table 17 shows that since 1977 the death rate has increased in the younger age groups but decreased in the older age groups, though since 1986 all age groups except the 30-39 year-olds have shown a decrease.

The figures also show that there were 22 per cent fewer deaths in women aged 50 and over in 1987 than there were in 1977, but deaths of women aged under 50 increased by 39 per cent over the same period.

One hopes that, despite the increase in positive smear rate, an improved national smear system will eventually bring the death even further down. The implementation of 'call and recall' systems in recent years by health authorities and doctors in Britain has clearly improved the uptake rate, as suggested by the figures in Table 13. In 1990, the government put the onus on doctors to chase patients to have their smears by setting them payment targets. The targets are related to the percentage of smears taken each year from the number of women on the practice list who are due for a smear. The aim is to encourage GPs to make sure that they have an efficient system for notifying women that they need a smear. The next couple of years will show whether this policy has improved the situation.

However, there is no statutory obligation on doctors to perform smears, so many women still have to come forward on their own initiative. This means that, unless there is a national or local publicity campaign to remind women of the dangers of cervical cancer, they can easily ignore the need for a smear.

The women most likely to be prompted are those young enough to be informed about smear testing when they visit family planning clinics, or middle aged women with access to information about cervical cancer. This does not include many of the high risk women who either do not attend a family planning clinic or who are not well educated in health care. As the 1980 'Black

Report' on social inequalities in health pointed out, women from social classes IV and V (the poorest classes) are far less likely to have smears than women from higher social classes while women from the lower social classes suffer a far higher mortality rate.

There are a number of reasons why women may miss a smear and these are more likely to affect the lower classes. Many such women have never had a smear, a repeat smear, or smears within a reasonably safe time period of each other. The fact that the vast majority of women in Britain who die from cervical cancer have never had a smear shows that the screening still needs to be better directed at the women who most need it. Interestingly, studies have shown that 90 per cent of women would respond to a call for a smear if they were approached properly. Such an approach has still to be worked out. Another problem in the past was that the government guidelines concentrated on screening women over 35. Yet a recent large study (carried out in a North London practice) published in the British Medical Journal (*BMJ*,1987, **294**, p.1326-1328), has shown that this policy did not take into account the younger women who may have cervical pre-cancer at a stage where it can be identified and cured. In the survey, over one year, of all the women who attended the colposcopy clinic (the first GP-based service in Britain) over half the early signs of the disease were spotted in the under-35s. The highest abnormality rate was in the 25-34 age group. Other large studies have also shown this. In 1990 the British government updated its recommendations to include taking smears on a five-yearly basis from women in the 25-64 age group. These recommendations are continually under review, as more epidemiological data comes to light.

Screening in the United States

Around 60,000 women a year are expected to develop cancer of the cervix, with around 7,000 women dying from the disease annually. This is an improvement on the previous three decades, during which time the cervical smear (or Pap smear as it is commonly known in the United States) has become one of the most common laboratory tests in the United States.

However, the American College of Obstetricians and Gynecologists has drawn attention to the high number of false-negative results, in the region of 20-40 per cent. This has occurred because of the nature of private medicine in the United States. A *Wall Street Journal* investigation revealed 'a picture of a Pap-screening industry kept afloat by over-worked, undersupervised, poorly paid technicians'. These technicians are often paid on a piecework basis, which critics say encourages then to rush the analysis.

In the past the American Cancer Society has recommended a Pap test every three years after two consecutive annual tests. However, the American College of Obstetricians and Gynecologists has been critical of this policy in view of the high rate of false-negative smears, which has been blamed on the failure of physicians to take adequate samples. It has also been suggested that laboratories are reluctant to reject 'inadequate smears', for fear of losing business.

Colposcopy

The British Society for Clinical Cytology (BSCC) recently recommended that all women with dyskaryotic cells in their smear, however mild, should be referred for colposcopy. It has only recently been recognized that mild abnormalities on smears can be falsely reassuring, as, in some cases, subsequent colposcopic examination shows that a more severe abnormality (CIN 3) exists within deeper layers of the cervical skin. The problem with the recommendation of the BSCC is that there are not enough colposcopes or colposcopists to cope with the large number of women whose cytology warrants colposcopic investigation.

The development of the author's colposcopy service has shown that colposcopy can be successfully performed outside of a hospital setting and as a leader in the *British Medical Journal* (*BMJ*, 1987, **294**, p.1307) put it, 'The development of such clinics may be not only desirable but vital.'

Chapter 14

Cases from the practice

THE MAJORITY OF WOMEN who present for a smear have their smear correctly interpreted, and any pre-cancer detected is almost always effectively treated. However, some of the case histories described below are of a type occasionally encountered in general practice and hospital situations and include examples where occasionally a woman is either failed by the system or by herself. These cases are included to help illustrate various points made in the text of this book and which we believe will be of interest to readers. It is important to make it clear that none of these cases actually represents any specific individual. However, any doctors describing imaginary cases will, of course, draw on their own personal experience and that of their patients.

Case one   Intercourse at an early age
Angela wanted to start sleeping with her boyfriend at the age of 16 and went to her GP for contraceptive advice. After preliminary explanations and check-up, which at that time did not include a vaginal examination, she chose, and was prescribed, the Pill. She attended her customary check-up a few months later, and a year later a cervical smear was taken. She had had only one boyfriend throughout that particular year and was still seeing him. The smear was reported as containing severely dyskaryotic cells. On colposcopic examination, a very large area of

abnormality on her cervix was seen. A biopsy showed extensive CIN 3.

A year ago, this girl was a virgin and she only had one boyfriend. Examination of the boyfriend did not reveal any genital warts, and he had previously had only one girlfriend. He thought that she may have had genital warts, but he wasn't sure. Angela had a laser evaporation of the abnormality on her cervix, which healed perfectly without leaving a trace of the disease.

Subsequent smears during the next three years were all normal. However, both she and her boyfriend continued to be anxious, and it took a long time and many consultations to persuade them that they couldn't blame themselves in any way and that the best thing they could possibly do was for Angela to have regular smears. Angela's fertility was unlikely to be affected because of her treatment.

It is, however, interesting to note that in Angela's case history, her mother had cervical cancer, and that there was also a history of breast cancer in the family. It would appear that Angela's immune and genetic make-up gave her a predisposition to this kind of problem. Angela fulfilled two other predisposing risk factors: she started intercourse at a very early age, before the transformation zone on the cervix had fully matured and thus it is possible that this lining was immature and as yet unready to defend itself, and she was a smoker, having started to smoke when she was 14 and she was smoking more than 10 cigarettes a day.

An interesting feature in this case is that, if one assumes that Angela's cervix was free of the disease before the onset of sexual intercourse, it took less than a year for her to develop a severe form of cervical pre-cancer. Furthermore, if she had been smeared much later, it may have been too late for local treatment and she may have needed an extensive cone biopsy or hysterectomy.

Case two   High risk male partner
Norma was 29, and had had only two partners. Her smears had always been normal. The most recent smear came a year after she had acquired her new partner. This was abnormal and showed mild dyskaryosis. A colposcopy was carried out and there was

a small area of abnormality on the cervix which, on biopsy, showed her to have CIN 3. It was still very superficial and was evaporated with a laser. The new lining regrew perfectly, the cervix appearing completely healed, and her subsequent smears for the next three years were normal. On further investigation into her partner's previous sexual partner, the following information came to light: her partner had been married twice before. His first wife died of cervical cancer, and his second wife subsequently developed the disease and was treated elsewhere (although we had few details of this), and Norma, his girlfriend had also developed the disease.

He left her for another woman but we felt we should inform him about the possibility that he may be a carrier of something which may induce the disease and thus pose a threat to his new girlfriend. It so happened that we were able to send for him to be examined and he was found to have genital warts. When these were sampled and analysed by the laboratory, the same wart virus was found in a genital wart on his penis as was found in the cervical pre-cancer of my patient.

By the time we gave him this information, his new girlfriend was found to have a dyskaryotic smear. Undoubtedly he represents a high risk male who seems to be transmitting some kind of agent capable of inducing the disease in his sexual partners. He was offered an explanation and advised to wear a sheath in order to protect his women partners in future.

The whole episode left my patient very embittered and very sad and she has as yet not been able to form a new relationship with anyone. Although we were able to eradicate her disease, she still felt herself to be at risk of recurrence. She also feels that she may infect any man she may subsequently make love to and, furthermore, she worried that such a man infected by her, will unknowingly induce cervical cancer to any subsequent sexual partners or indeed give it back to her. She felt very guilty about this despite the fact that she has been offered a full explanation and is a bright and extremely intelligent woman.

Case three   Post-menopausal woman in a second marriage
Beryl was a 65-year-old whose husband was killed ten years ago

in a car crash. Her previous smear, performed about six years ago was reported as normal. She remarried three years later and her husband was a widower.

She came to register at the surgery and did not request a cervical smear at all. She was very surprised when it was suggested she had one, because she thought she would be unlikely to develop cervical cancer at her age. However, she was persuaded to have a smear which was reported as inflammatory. On the basis of this, a colposcopy was performed and evidence of abnormality was found which was biopsied and shown to be CIN 3. The top of the abnormality could not be seen clearly, and on referral to hospital, this lady had a cone biopsy. Histology of the cone showed that she had carcinoma *in situ* which was still confined in the cervical canal. The histological report revealed that the cone biopsy had been a diagnosis and treatment in one, as the carcinoma *in situ* did not extend beyond the margin of the cone and was thus completely cut out. We don't know how long she had this disease, whether it was from the first or second husband. The second was examined for genital warts and none were found.

In this case, the fact that she had not had a smear for over five years, that the previous smear was normal, and that her latest smear did not show any abnormal cells apart from mild inflammation shows that even a mild abnormality at post-menopausal age should be considered as a potential malignancy. The fact that she had acquired a new partner was also significant.

The case demonstrates also the need to sample adequately the endocervical canal where a disease may hide beyond the reach of a standard spatula.

There are instances of some women in whom sampling from the cervical canal is extremely difficult. These cases include post-menopausal women and women who have had operations on their cervices resulting in stenosis of the cervical canal. These women may have to be examined by colposcope and their smear taken under colposcopic surveillance. Sampling from some post-menopausal women may need up to ten day's pre-treatment with oestrogen prior to a smear. Oestrogens will activate the cervical linings to become accessible to good smear taking.

Beryl's follow-up smears for the last years were normal. Cone biopsy proved to be both diagnostic and curative, saving her from major surgery such as a hysterectomy. However, the prime means of detection was the cervical smear.

Case four   Post-natal check-up

Wanda, a social worker, was thirty-six years old when she had her third baby. Her smear taken during pregnancy was reported as normal. Six weeks after the baby was born, she came for a post-natal check-up and contraceptive advice and it was at that time that I noticed, even with the naked eye, a thick white skin on an area of her cervix, suggesting a possible pre-cancer. She was colposcoped and the abnormality biopsied. Histology of the biopsy confirmed the presence of CIN 3 and Wanda had laser treatment which cleared the disease completely. On re-checking the smear taken during Wanda's pregnancy, there were no abnormal cells to be seen. The cellular content on the slide was adequate, and yet the pre-cancer must have existed during pregnancy because it is very unlikely that CIN 3 could have developed in a normal cervical skin in such a short period of time. It may have been that the spatula had missed the pre-cancer during smear taking, or pre-cancer cells did not come away easily. If Wanda had had a repeat smear at the age of forty, as suggested by the government guidelines at the time, it is likely that there may have been a serious progression of the undetected disease, possibly to invasive cancer.

Case five   CIN and pre-conceptual counselling

Mary was a 30-year-old teacher who had been divorced and had recently married again. She wanted to have a baby and attended a pre-conceptual counselling check-up which included a smear. The cytologist's report revealed a mild to moderate dyskaryosis. Without waiting for the result, Mary moved away without leaving details of her new address, and it took quite an extensive investigation to find that she and her husband had gone abroad. We finally traced her and the result was conveyed. She was at that time abroad and she went to a local professor of gynaecology who took another smear and inspected her cervix and told her that he did not see any abnormality. Her smear came back as normal. He advised her that there were no visible cervical abnormalities and if she wanted to have a baby she could go ahead. Nevertheless, she doubted his opinion and returned to England for colposcopy, even though her second smear was normal. The colposcopy revealed an area of abnormality deep in the canal and when that area was biopsied, it was shown to be a carcinoma *in situ*. The abnormality was successfully treated with a laser. The cervix healed perfectly and her follow-up colposcopy and smear were normal. She became pregnant within six months of the treatment and had a normal delivery of a healthy baby girl. Further smears combined with colposcopy proved normal.

The case demonstrates the need for both the woman and the person taking the smear to agree that they need to contact each other with the results. The patient should be made aware that if she changes address then she must tell the centre where she had her smear taken. The case also demonstrates that a normal smear following a recent abnormal one should be viewed with caution and should be followed by colposcopy if possible. Furthermore, pre-conceptual check-up is an excellent opportunity for a woman to have a smear and thus to safeguard herself against the problem of pre-cancer occuring during pregnancy, at which time the treatment should be avoided because of the risk of inducing miscarriage. The above case also shows how, after local treatment for cervical pre-cancer, the cervix usually heals well and fertility is unaffected.

If the condition had not been identified and treated and she had become pregnant, the disease might have advanced and eventually proved a threat to her fertility and even her life.

Case six False-negative smear result

Eileen, a married 60-year-old housewife, had a routine health check-up which included a cervical smear. This was her first smear after an interval of five years. The smear was reported as normal. No future recall was suggested. She subsequently attended her GP a year later for reasons unconnected with any cervical cytology but was persuaded to have another smear as a routine check and this time the smear revealed a few mildly dyskaryotic cells. She was colposcoped and the colposcopic biopsy showed a microinvasive carcinoma which required a cone biopsy. During the cone biopsy Eileen started to bleed uncontrollably and in order to stop the bleeding the surgeon had to proceed to a vaginal hysterectomy. It later transpired that, unknown to her surgeon, Eileen had been taking large doses of aspirin for her arthritis which has a side effect of increased bleeding. She had never mentioned this to her surgeon.

Such complications rarely happen but underline the importance of a patient giving their doctor a full history, however unimportant a small detail might seem to be, such as the taking of aspirin in this instance.

In the four years since the operation, all her vault smears taken under colposcopic examination have been absolutely normal and she is fit and well. However on going back and checking her so-called 'normal' smear from the year before her abnormal one, it was shown that a few inflammatory and possibly dyskaryotic cells were present on the slide but had been missed and not reported. Thus a disease in a post-menopausal woman may be missed and it is advisable to continue to perform smears at realistic intervals.

Case seven   New partner—new disease

Janet, a 41-year-old woman was widowed and left with two children. Three years later she married a long distance lorry driver whose first wife had died of cervical cancer. Prior to Janet's second marriage she had always had regular smears which were reported as normal.

Within a year of re-marriage she had a smear which was reported as mildly dyskaryotic. However, colposcopic biopsy showed the disease to be more severe, in fact CIN 3, and she required a cone biopsy which showed an invasive carcinoma and she finally had a hysterectomy. She remained free of the disease and the follow-up for the last four years has shown her to be free of the disease.

In view of the fact that all her previous smears had been normal and became abnormal only on subsequent remarriage, it would appear that her new husband may have played some role in inducing the disease. The evidence shows that behavioural and occupational characteristics of one's sexual partner may be a predisposing factor to cervical cancer. Statistics show that long-distance lorry drivers' wives have been found to have a greater incidence of this disease. As Janet's new husband was in a high risk category as regards his occupation, it is possible that her change of husband put her at greater risk of cervical cancer. He may have picked up (and possibly induced) a sexually transmitted factor such as HPV from previous partners which subsequently contributed to the induction of Janet's cancer.

Case eight *Cervical pre-cancer and pregnancy*

Sheila was a 26-year-old housewife with one child. She had always had normal smears, but a recent smear revealed mild dyskaryosis. Colposcopy identified an abnormal area which the biopsy showed to be CIN 3. Before local treatment could be organized, Sheila was found to be pregnant (in fact, she must have been pregnant at the time of the biopsy). An ultrasound scan showed her to be carrying twins. The treatment of CIN had to be postponed. Her cervix was observed colposcopically during pregnancy during which time the disease did not progress. Sheila had a normal vaginal delivery of a healthy son and daughter. Colposcopy at the six weeks post-natal check showed no abnormality on her cervix and the smear was normal. One year later, Sheila's smear was again mildly dyskaryotic, the biopsy showed CIN 3 again, and she had laser treatment. The following three annual smears were normal.

This case illustrates several interesting points. Firstly, although the cervical smear is the prime indicator of a cervical abnormality it failed to reveal the degree of abnormality as shown by colposcopy and biopsy. The assessment of the disease and its progression potential would not have been accurate when using the smear only as a guide. Secondly, although the abnormality seemed to disappear after the delivery (as suggested by smears and colposcopy), it was possible that there was some residual disease or simply that a new abnormality had developed. In this case, a severe dyskaryosis developed within a year, and, prior to that, a mild degree of abnormality on a smear did not reveal an underlying severe disease.

During the last year I have had more than ten women in whom abnormal, or pre-cancerous or cancerous cells have been diagnosed right at the onset of their pregnancy. The colposcopic examinations showed them to have areas of abnormality varying from CIN 1 to CIN 3. In all the cases, the top of the lesion could clearly be seen but, of course, a more accurate estimate of the depth into which this disorder reached could have been better diagnosed by taking a good biopsy. However, taking biopsies from pregnant cervices can be very risky. There may be bleeding from the cervix which is very rich in blood vessels. If an adequate biopsy is not taken, there may be a risk of missing a more advanced form of the disease, such as an invasive cancer which could become more disseminated. Biopsies may need to be taken when a colposcopist suspects invasion or when colposcopy is not available and biopsy may be the only diagnostic procedure with which to follow-up a severely abnormal smear. It is advisable to have a normal smear reported before starting pregnancy, especially nowadays when older women are having babies for the first time and have had many years of sexual activity and more partners than younger women, thus putting them at greater risk of developing a pre-cancer.

Case nine   Lena—a case of mistaken faith
Lena was a 30-year-old who desparately wanted a child but had difficulty conceiving. After a suggestion by a friend, she went to a homoeopath. When she eventually had a baby she was convinced that the homoeopath's treatment had been helpful. At the time she lived abroad, and, after her husband got a job in London, she came to the practice to register, when she was offered a cervical smear. Whilst taking the smear the practice nurse observed a small white area on her cervix and called me in. This area looked very suspicious and Lena was offered colposcopy on the spot. This revealed an area which looked like a carcinoma *in situ* and a biopsy was duly taken, and the diagnosis was confirmed. Lena was offered a thorough explanation that urgent treatment was needed, and an appointment was made for her to attend the local hospital colposcopy clinic for laser treatment of the abnormal area. The nature and seriousness of her condi-

tion was fully explained along with how laser treatment offered the safe possibility of complete eradication of the disease. Two weeks later she failed to turn up for her appointment, did not answer any of the subsequent letters and was always out when we telephoned.

Three months later Lena turned up at the surgery and pronounced triumphantly that she was 'cured' and now had no symptoms whatsoever. (She had forgotten that she had never had any signs or symptoms before or after her original smear.) Now she had come for confirmation that everything was cured. The reason for Lena's supposed miraculous cure was that she had been to the same homoeopath who had helped her previously, and he had given her some pills and assurances that the disease would be cured. She explained that she failed to turn up for her laser treatment because she had faith that her homoeopath would cure her. She also told us that she had been frightened, believing that hospital treatment would prevent future pregnancies, and she was keen to have more children. This fear continued in spite of the verbal and written assurances given at her first consultation that laser treatment was very unlikely to impair future pregnancies. She was colposcoped during her visit and the present abnormality was compared to notes of its previous descriptions. The abnormal area had literally quadrupled in size. It was explained to Lena as gently as possible, that the homoeopathic treatment had not managed to remove the disease, and that it had progressed, hopefully not too far for laser treatment. I persuaded her that hospital treatment was essential and Lena had a small cone biopsy by laser shortly afterwards. Fortunately, the cone biopsy was reported as having removed the whole of the carcinoma *in situ*. The cervix healed normally and Lena is now hoping to become pregnant again.

Case ten *Cost of a smear — a life*

Jackie was 25 when she had her first son. Two years later she was divorced from her husband and left to bring up her son alone. She took a job in a nearby pub as a barmaid and around the same time acquired a new boyfriend. Jackie subsequently attended the local family planning clinic for contraceptive advice.

She was not given a smear at that time because she thought she had had one at the time of her son's birth two years previously. When she asked her GP for a smear two years later, he refused, on the grounds that five years had not yet elapsed since her last one, referring to what was at that time the government's recommended time gap between smears. Finally, when she was thirty years old she was given a smear which proved to be abnormal and she was recalled for a repeat smear. That smear also proved to be abnormal, although due to a mix-up with sending the result she only discovered it by phoning the clinic some months later.

Her GP referred her to a colposcopy clinic where she had to wait six weeks for an appointment. During that time she began to suffer from very bad backache and a dragging sensation along both sides of her legs. She also noticed an occasional blood-stained discharge after sex. When she was seen at the colposcopy clinic she was told that she would have to have a cone biopsy immediately.

Unfortunately, the cone biopsy showed an invasive cancer and Jackie's stay of a few days turned out to be much longer, as she had to have a total hysterectomy. At the operation, several lymph glands in her pelvis, abdomen, and even right up in her diaphragm were found to be taken up by the cancer cells. Tragically, Jackie died six months later. On investigation, it was discovered that she did not have a cervical smear but a high vaginal swab during her pregnancy. As she never received any results she assumed all was well.

This case shows how important it is to know for sure whether a smear or high vaginal swab has been taken and to find out the results of the tests. Furthermore, the fact that she was in a new sexual relationship meant that she should have had another smear but her request was rejected by her GP who pointed to the five-yearly screening policy which existed in that area. The smear, when it did come, was too late as were her signs and symptoms. Ironically, she lived in an area where the facilities existed to save her life, but the system failed her.

Case eleven   Smears in a post-hysterectomy woman
Mrs Naraini was a delightful Hindu housewife married and in

her early fifties. She had had four pregnancies and on her fifth one bled very badly and had to be rushed for an emergency hysterectomy at a local hospital near where she was living in India. She made a full recovery and for the next six years she was fit and well and did not need to see her doctor during this period. It was also at this time that she moved to London. She came to the practice after she developed a slight blood-stained discharge. On examination, a high vaginal vault smear was taken and the cytological report showed it to contain severely dyskaryotic cells. Mrs Naraini was colposcoped and areas of abnormality were seen in the vaginal vault (her cervix had been removed by the hysterectomy), that is the top of the skin of the vagina, left behind after the cervix and uterus had been removed.

Biopsies of the abnormal area showed a squamous cell carcinoma even though Mrs Naraini's cervix had been removed. There was also a form of pre-cancer of the vaginal wall called a vaginal intraepithelial neoplasia (VAIN), occuring in the place where the top of the vagina must have been detached from the uterus during hysterectomy. Mrs Naraini had to have many painful repetitive treatments by laser and radiotherapy to try to prevent the spread of the malignancy.

Had she been properly checked at the time of her hysterectomy it might have been possible to identify the pre-cancer/cancer in her cervix at the time of her hysterectomy and to have removed the diseased tissue in its entirety.

Prior to her hysterectomy, Mrs Naraini did not have a cervical smear and it is likely that hysterectomy was carried out in ignorance of any cervical abnormality, and failed to remove some abnormal areas of the vagina and vaginal skin portion covering the cervix. Pre-cancerous or cancerous cells were left behind in the remaining vaginal vault. Had Mrs Naraini attended regularly for smears, her disease would have been detected much earlier. This case demonstrates the importance of having regular smears, especially before hysterectomy. After such an operation it is important to have smears on a regular basis. There should also be a histological analysis of the cervix removed at hysterectomy for other reasons than malignancy (such as uterine fibroids or pregnancy emergency) because a previously undiagnosed cervical malignancy may be identified and suggest the possibility of its spread to some of the remaining tissues left after surgery.

Where pre-cancer or cancer exists, colposcopy before and after surgery increases the chance of detection and treatment to prevent further malignancy.

Case twelve   The 'guilty' mistress?

Lynette was a bubbly 26-year-old clerk in a bank who began having an affair with a married colleague. Soon after starting the affair with him she developed genital herpes. He denied having the disease. Lynette's herpetic spots on her vulva and vagina soon disappeared, and very soon afterwards she became pregnant. She decided to continue with the pregnancy and at the antenatal clinic she had a cervical smear which was reported on as mildly abnormal. A repeat smear was recommended. Lynette became very frightened — she thought she may be harbouring cervical cancer. She had heard that herpes was thought to cause cervical cancer although there is now little evidence for this. She was worried that her smear may have missed an underlying, more severe form of the disease and she was also worried that she may have transmitted herpes to her boss who in turn may have infected his wife putting her at risk of cervical cancer!

She took her problems to a private gynaecologist and had colposcopy which did not show any evidence of pre-cancer, and a further smear and high vaginal swab showed only a mild thrush (an infection common in pregnancy). He further explained to her that there is little evidence to connect herpes with cervical cancer. Much relieved by the explanation, Lynette went on to have a normal delivery of a baby boy. Regular smears after the delivery were normal. However, she begged her partner to persuade his wife to have a cervical smear and a test for herpes.

The wife did go for a smear, not because her husband thought it was a good idea, but as a result of a national campaign poster recommending smears which she saw in a local health centre while taking a friend to the doctors. On subsequent medical examination, there was no evidence of genital herpes but she was found to have a severely dyskaryotic smear and after colposcopy and biopsy she had laser treatment which removed the pre-cancer completely. In the light of her experience, the wife then wrote to her mother who at that time was living in Paris and was in her late fifties, and advised her to have a smear. The mother felt that there was no need to go, and protested that she was no longer sexually active and had never been promiscuous, and thus she did not need a smear. However, her daughter was adamant and took her to have a smear, which was abnormal. Colposcopy showed a small area of pre-cancer, deep in the cervical canal but still quite visible in its entirety. The pre-cancer was successfully treated and follow-up smears on both mother and daughter were normal, but Lynette felt she was in some way to blame for the onset of the pre-cancer in the first place.

The case highlights the problems of guilt and confusion that can exist in love affairs involving a third party, particularly as it is unlikely that Lynette had anything to do with the pre-cancer which appeared in his wife. It was more likely to be a coincidence. It can be a very harrowing experience to tell one's sexual partner that they should seek urgent medical advice for a condition they may have acquired by picking up a sexually transmitted cancer-inducing agent from their other lover. However, unless these people are made aware of the possibility that they may be harbouring a pre-cancerous condition which can be detected and cured, the long-term outcome may be far worse than just hurt feelings. The case also shows the need to have smears and follow-up investigations at any time in one's life, as the only way it will make itself known in its early stages is on a smear. It also shows that by persuading women to have smears, their lives can be saved.

Case thirteen   False sense of security
Isabel was a 26-year-old teacher married to an oil rig engineer. She had a smear at a local family planning clinic and was told that she would be informed of the result if it was positive. Two months later Isabel and her husband moved to a new house in another part of town and after another couple of months settling in their new home they registered with me. Isabel was offered a cervical smear but declined as she had had a normal smear

four months previously. Because her husband was going to work on an oil rig in Saudi Arabia, she no longer needed any contraception, and thus had no internal examination. They planned to start a family after his return. Two months after her registration, Isabel's previous medical records had arrived. On checking these, a cervical smear reporting severely dyskaryotic cells was found in the notes.

The smear had been taken six months previously and had not been followed up. I recalled Isabel, took another smear, and then had to rush her into hospital where the disease was found to be so advanced as to require a hysterectomy. This was a tragedy for, at 26, Isabel was well in every other respect and hoped and planned to have children. On investigation it was found that the report on an abnormal smear arrived at the family planning clinic long after Isabel had moved away. The smear took a little longer to process as is sometimes the case with abnormal smears because they are usually scrutinized by as many as three cytologists if an abnormality is supected. The clinic tried to contact Isabel but failed. They also informed her previous GP who tried to contact Isabel, but he had no forwarding address.

Isabel did not enquire for her result because she was told that she would be contacted only if there was something wrong. As she had heard nothing within two months of the smear, after which she moved house, she assumed that her smear was normal. She did not think of informing her GP or family planning clinic of her new address and did not arrange with the post office to redirect her mail.

The system of informing women only of positive results, lulled Isabel into believing that her smear was normal, nearly cost her her life, and tragically lost her the chance of giving birth to a child. As it was, she was lucky her old records were checked and the abnormal report found, otherwise her positive result could have been missed altogether, and, by the time she would have had another smear, the disease may have become untreatable.

By either telephoning the clinic or informing her GP of a change of address or getting the post office to re-direct her mail, Isabel could have ensured that her result would have reached her and the six months of blissful ignorance and delay while the pre-cancer was growing, may just possibly have made the difference between local treatment and a hysterectomy.

Case fourteen   You're never too old for a smear

Maria was 76 and had been a widow for the last ten years and had never had a smear. Recently, she visited her GP on numerous occasions, complaining of a backache and constipation and lately reported that she thought she had seen some blood in her bowel motion. The GP did not examine her but did prescribe some laxatives, suppositories, and pain relievers. None of these worked and Maria continued to have pain. Finally, she sought a second opinion and, on vaginal examination, which was difficult because of vaginal narrowing due to age, and she was found to have a mass fixed to the top of her vagina which bled when it was touched.

The mass was undoubtedly due to cervical carcinoma and a smear taken from it confirmed the presence of very malignant cells. Pelvic X-rays and ultrasound in hospital showed the presence of a mass in the pelvis invading the bowel. She was found to have Stage IV (the most severe form) cervical cancer and she was offered radiotherapy as the disease had gone beyond the stage where surgery would have been effective. Regular smearing would almost certainly have detected the disease in its early curative stage, enabling timely intervention and avoidance of suffering.

Case fifteen   Will I ever be cured?

Lynn, a 30-year-old married teacher with two children, had a smear reported as as being mildly dyskaryotic. Colposcopy showed that there was a large area on her cervix which needed treatment and this was done at the local hospital using diathermy, the only treatment available there at the time.

Following treatment, the cervix healed well and for the next two years follow-up smears were reported on as normal. However, in the third, colposcopy following another mildly dyskaryotic smear result revealed a very small area of abnormality which needed to be treated. By this time, the local hospital had acquired a laser machine and treatment was performed on an out-patient basis, resulting in eradication of the abnormality.

Shortly after her second treatment, Lynn became pregnant

and had her third child quite normally. A smear after the delivery was reported on as normal, but a year later, Lynn once again had a mildly dyskaryotic smear, and biopsy showed a CIN 3, and she required yet another treatment by laser. By this time, both Lynn and her husband were quite distressed by this, both stating that they had been faithful to each other, and that every time Lynn had her treatment she had been assured by doctors of a 95 per cent cure rate, yet here was this recurrence. Neither she nor her husband could understand why she could not have been cured once and for all, why the abnormality kept recurring and what the use was of having all these smears and treatment.

No-one is to blame for such recurrence, but the need for regular screening and treatment where necessary cannot be emphasized enough. The ease and effectiveness of modern treatments means that they should not be feared.

Chapter 15

Questions and answers

What causes cervical cancer?
The most common form (squamous cell carcinoma) of cervical
pre-cancer and cancer is thought to be instigated by chemical,
bacterial or viral agent(s) transmitted during sexual intercourse.
Evidence points to certain varieties of the human papilloma virus
as being involved but there may be other factors involved such
as genetics and immunity. For example, a much rarer form of
cervical cancer known as adenocarcinoma, has been observed
in virgins (who never suffer from squamous cell cancer). This
means that sexual intercourse is not the only cause.

How soon after sexual intercourse can this disease develop?
It is impossible to put a definite time scale on the development
or rate of progression of the disease. The first appearance of pre-
cancerous change in the cells of the cervical skin can appear in
as little as a few months or may take years to develop. These
changes can only be detected by taking a cervical smear. However,
it may take many years for such changes or signs as bleeding
or discharge to develop. Because of this potentially huge and variable time lag, it is often impossible to blame any one partner
for causing the disease. As the disease takes time to develop and
progress into more severe forms, having a smear within a year
of first intercourse with a new partner can detect the beginnings
of an abnormality which can then be removed.

What is CIN?

This term stands for cervical intraepithelial neoplasia, the name given to a pre-cancerous change in the cells still confined to the skin in the cervix.

Are there any signs or symptoms of CIN?

Usually there are none, but on rare occasions there may be post-coital bleeding or discharge. These are more commonly present at the advanced stages of cervical cancer.

How can CIN be detected?

By having a cervical smear.

What is involved in having a cervical smear taken?

It involves visiting a doctor or nurse trained to take smears. This may be at a surgery, hospital, family planning or well-woman clinic. It is best to avoid having a smear during menstruation, and the best time to attend is during mid-cycle. The entire procedure is usually completely painless. You will be asked to remove your underwear, lie on a couch with your knees bent and slightly apart. A speculum is inserted into the vagina which opens it and reveals the cervix and the vaginal walls. The smear is taken using a special instrument known as a cervical spatula which is rotated and scrapes off the cells lining the cervix. The cells are then spread on to a glass slide which is immediately flooded with fixative. The slide should bear your name, date of smear being taken, and your date of birth. Appropriate forms should be filled in to include details such as contraceptive measures, all previous pregnancies, results of previous smears and treatments.

How do I get the results of my smear?

There is a great variety of methods used by different centres to inform women about their results. Many centres inform patients only if their result is abnormal, while others ask you to telephone for your result. The most satisfactory approach is the one where every result, positive or negative, is sent in writing to the patient, explaining the result and enclosing the next suggested date for re-screening. There have been instances of women being lulled into a false sense of security by not receiving a result and assuming their smear was normal. Deaths have occurred because the positive result may have got lost somewhere along the line of administration or even in the post. Sometimes there may even be a failure to notify a change of address or the notifying centre may have taken it down wrongly. Make sure you give a correct address and update it if you move. *Do not assume that your result is normal.* If you are not notified about it, be sure to enquire. In an imperfect world, make yourself responsible for finding out the result.

What does it mean if I have an abnormal smear?
This is when the cytologist has seen and reported any kind of an abnormal cell on the smear slide. *An abnormal smear does not necessarily mean that there is a cancer present or that the cells are pre-cancerous*—they may be inflammatory cells which may revert to normal or they may look abnormal as a result of infection. The next step should be to have further investigation by repeat smear and/or colposcopy.

What is a normal or negative smear?
One where there is no visual evidence of cellular abnormality.

What is an inadequate smear?
Where there are too few cells on the slide, or endocervical cells are missing, or the smear cells are obscured by discharge. Cytologists may also call this a 'scanty smear'. In such circumstances the smear should be repeated.

What is a positive smear?
One containing cells which have been reported as being dyskaryotic, i.e. having such a variable degree of nuclear disturbance as to suggest that a pre-cancerous or even cancerous change is taking place on the cervix. Internationally a positive smear is regarded as a severely dyskaryotic one and regarded as equivalent to CIN 3 or more. All women with a dyskaryotic result should have colposcopy.

What happens next if I have an abnormal or positive smear?
Depending on the cytologist's report, either a repeat smear is suggested or a colposcopy examination is recommended.

Why do I need a repeat smear?
A repeat smear is needed when the previous smear was either reported as being inadequate (too few cells on the slide), or having an abnormality which may be very mild and might go away in time, but which must be followed up for safety. If an abnormality is thought to be caused by a bacterial or fungal infection, for example, then the infection must be identified, treated, and cleared up. The smear should then be repeated to check whether treatment has indeed cleared the abnormality. If the abnormality persists, colposcopy may be recommended.

Why do I need colposcopy?
Colposcopy is used to investigate and follow up abnormalities on the cervix as detected by a cervical smear, or where a history of suspected disease exists despite a normal smear. Colposcopy may confirm the presence and spread of such abnormalities. If abnormalities are confirmed, further investigation using biopsy or cone biopsy may be necessary to determine appropriate treatment.

What is a punch biopsy and why do I need it?
A punch biopsy is a small piece of tissue taken from an abnormal area under colposcopic surveillance using biopsy forceps. The tissue is sent for histological examination in order to identify the nature and extent of abnormality more precisely. Such information allows doctors to assess whether and what kind of treatment is necessary.

What is the difference between a punch biopsy and a cone biopsy?
A punch biopsy removes a small piece of tissue and, because it is virtually painless, no anaesthetic is needed. A cone biopsy requires removal of a larger part of the cervix, usually under local or general anaesthetic.

I had a positive smear, but nothing abnormal was seen on colposcopy and biopsy. A repeat smear was again positive. Now I am told that I need a cone biopsy. As no abnormalities were found on colposcopy and biopsy, why do I need a cone biopsy?
A cone biopsy is indicated when colposcopy and biopsy fail to locate the source of the abnormal cells found on the cervical

smear. This can happen because the abnormal area may be too small to be identified by the magnification of the colposcope or may be in the cervical canal, beyond the vision of the colposcope. It may be that a few abnormal cells from it had drifted down on to the cervix and been picked up by a cervical smear. To investigate further, a cone biopsy is needed, where a larger piece of tissue is cut out in the shape of a cone and subsequently analysed by a histologist. Often the entire abnormal area is removed by the cone biopsy but if the abnormality extends to the edges of the cone, then more tissue must be removed, and a hysterectomy may be necessary. Occasionally, a cone biopsy is needed when an ordinary biopsy suggests the possibility of a more advanced disease and more tissue removal is needed to make a diagnosis of the spread and nature of the disease.

Which part of the cervix is likely to be affected by an abnormality?
The transformation zone (TZ) is the area on the cervix in which a change from endocervical to squamous epithelium takes place at the meeting point (squamocolumnar junction) of the two types of tissues. It is in this area that the abnormality is most likely to develop. Occasionally this area is found inside the endocervical canal—this often occurs after menopause or sometimes after operations for cervical pre-cancer, e.g. cone biopsy, laser or diathermy treatment.

If I have an early stage cervical cancer, how do I know that I have it?
There may be no signs or symptoms at all until the cancer becomes invasive. The only way to be sure of detecting cancer in its pre-cancerous and curable state is to have regular cervical smears.

What are the signs or symptoms which occasionally occur if a pre-cancer or cancer is present?
The presence of a pre-cancer does not usually manifest itself with any signs or symptoms. However, if the disease has progressed into a cancerous stage, and occasionally in the pre-cancerous stage, there are some tell-tale signs that all is not well with the cervix. These include: irregular bleeding or discomfort during or after intercourse; unusual vaginal discharge; pelvic pain;

swollen legs; and backache. Often these signs have nothing to do with cervical cancer, but a smear is essential to exclude this as a possibility. It is advisable to have a smear following any incidence of post-coital, post-menopausal or irregular bleeding (that is, between periods).

If I have contracted this disease and if I now make love with another boyfriend, am I likely to 'infect' him with whatever it is that has 'infected' me?
It is quite possible that you may infect him. There is evidence which shows that, if a man has intercourse with a woman suffering from cervical cancer or pre-cancer, it is more likely that his subsequent partners will also develop the disease. The use of a condom could protect the man in this instance.

How will I know that my husband or boyfriend is likely to transmit or give me this disease? How can I recognize it on him?
Genital warts are a sign that a man may transmit the disease. Not all these warts carry malignant potential, but evidence suggests that some warts contain the types of viruses which are thought to play a part in causing cervical cancer. Because tests for these are complicated and expensive, it is safer to assume that presence of genital warts in either partner does carry a high risk of women developing cervical cancer.

What does the human papilloma virus do and does it cause cancer?
It is not known what the role of HPV in cervical pre-cancer and cancer is. Recent studies have confirmed that some types of wart virus, which are contained in genital warts, have been found to be integrated in cells of pre-cancerous and cancerous tissues. It is likely that the virus is transmitted to the cervical tissue during sexual intercourse.

Do men with genital warts develop cancer on their penis?
Generally, no. Cancer of the penis is very rare. Most genital warts on men do not cause them to have penile cancer. A possible reason that the wart virus may pose a greater threat to women than men is that the virus may have a preference for infecting and causing cancerous change in the type of skin found on the cervix. Nevertheless, men with penile cancer do tend to have geni-

tal warts and women whose partners have had penile cancer seem to be at a greater risk of developing cervical cancer themselves.

If I have genital warts am I likely to develop cervical cancer?
If you have genital warts, you are at greater risk of developing cervical pre-cancers or cancers than a woman who has not got them, but early detection of a cervical abnormality and its subsequent removal is possible by having regular cervical smears.

How can I find out if I am a carrier of a wart virus and whether it is of a type associated with cervical cancer?
A cervical smear can suggest the presence of wart virus infection because of the presence of koilocytes, the hallmark of wart virus infection, where cells on the smear have a halo around their nucleus which has darkened and changed in appearance compared to normal. There are other tests which can identify the presence of wart virus and its specific type in the cells collected from the cervix and vagina. At present, these tests are time consuming and expensive and are confined to a few research centres. Radioactive materials are needed in the process of testing for the virus using a technique known as *DNA/DNA hybridization*. Ongoing research makes it more likely that such tests and newer tests will become cheaper, easier to perform, more widespread, and will probably be performed without the need for radioactive materials.

Are some men more likely to induce cervical cancer than others?
Yes. There are a number of predisposing factors which have been shown to relate to cervical cancer. They include occupation (usually heavy physical or industrial work), sexual behaviour characteristics (including contact with multiple partners and those who have had the disease), smoking, presence of genital warts and a history of previous female partners with cervical pre-cancer or cancer.

Are some women more susceptible to cervical cancer than others?
Yes. As in the answer to the last question, there are several predisposing factors similar to those for men which increase a woman's likelihood of developing cervical cancer. They include sexual behaviour (i.e. multiple partners), smoking, genetic sus-

ceptibility, such as low immunity against infection, early age of first intercourse, multiple pregnancies, low social class, use of narcotics and immunosuppressive drugs. As women get older their immunity decreases and this probably makes them more susceptible to cervical cancer.

How can I find out if my partner is likely to transmit a wart virus infection to me even though he has no genital warts on him?
If a man has a history of partners who have genital warts, it makes him a suspect as a carrier of the wart virus. It is possible for a man to be a carrier even if there is no evidence of penile warts. By colposcoping the penis and applying acetic acid, it may be possible to reveal possible areas of wart virus infection and to take smears for subsequent laboratory analysis to detect the virus. This screening is rarely performed as colposcopic facilities are usually too tied up with looking at more acute cervical abnormalities.

Can wart virus infection be treated?
Beyond the removal of visible warts, there is as yet no effective treatment to get rid of the virus. However, research into anti-viral drugs is promising. There are some anti-viral creams, tablets and paints which can be used to treat warts.

Should intercourse be avoided if I already have cervical cancer?
It all depends on the state of the disease, and you should follow the advice given by your own doctor. However, in general, if you only have a mild pre-cancer, intercourse can continue as usual but the male partner should wear a condom to protect himself from infection (although he may well be infected already) and possibly to protect the cervix from further damage from seminal contents.

How can we protect ourselves from cervical cancer?
By beginning one's sexual life later (early 20s), limiting the number of sexual partners during one's life, and having monogamous relationships and using barrier methods of contraception, particularly condoms. Other ways are by stopping smoking (of either or both partners); having good genital hygiene; and undergoing regular cervical smears to detect the disease in its early pre-

cancerous stage and enable prevention of its progression to an invasive cancer by prompt removal of diseased tissue.

Does the Pill increase the chance of getting cervical cancer?
It has long been shown that long-term Pill users are more likely to acquire this disease. Many suggestions have been put forward to explain why this should be. Some include the fact that since the Pill is used there is no barrier method of contraception, therefore the cervix is left exposed to possible seeding for infection by agents in the semen. However, evidence that the Pill may have an active role to play comes from a study (by the Family Planning Association and Oxford University) which compared Pill users with IUD (intrauterine device or coil) users. There was an increasing risk associated with duration of Pill-taking compared to IUD users. After eight years use, the risk was two to three times greater than that of IUD users. However, this did not take into account their sexual behaviour characteristics and therefore the risk assessment may not necessarily be a reflection of the effect of the Pill.

What is the point of treating me if my partner is going to re-infect me again?
The first and most important thing to do is to be cleared of the existing abnormality because if you are not treated for a pre-cancer, the chances are that the disease may progress and become life-threatening. In clearing the disease, the entire transformation zone of the cervix where the abnormal area is situated is destroyed, and the new lining which re-grows and covers the neck of the womb is less likely to become cancerous, even if intercourse continues with the same partner. Nevertheless, the chance of the disease occurring again still exists. As the disease takes some time to develop, if a woman is reinfected by her partner, any pre-cancerous change will be picked up on subsequent smears, which should be performed annually. If there is a recurrence, it can be treated and re-treated in the same way as before.

If my boyfriend has been found to have a penile wart, should he be treated?
Penile warts should be treated because present evidence suggests

a link between wart virus and cervical cancer. The nature of this association is not yet clear.

Why doesn't my boyfriend develop penile cancer if he is infected with HPV?
A cancer of the penis is a rare condition. HPV is suspected of being involved in instigating a pre-cancer only on a particular type of skin which is predominantly the transformation zone on the cervix. In cases of penile cancer which are very rare HPV does seem to be implicated.

How are penile warts treated?
Treatment involves removal of the warts. This is accomplished by painting them with corrosive substances such as podophyllin or freezing them off (cryotherapy), burning them off (diathermy) or cutting them out (knife or laser). Method of treatment is usually dictated by the size of the wart and what facilities are available. The above treatments do not guarantee the eradication of wart virus from the genital tract and it may exist without manifestation as warts. Sometimes persistent attempts succeed in inducing an immune response which gets rid of warts and the virus completely.

Is it possible to remove the virus completely from the female genital tract?
One can never be sure that any infectious agent has been removed from the body in its entirety. All that can be said is that an area has been removed in which a virus or viruses or infections have expressed themselves by inducing a pre-cancerous or cancerous state. The infectious agent may be hiding elsewhere in the genital tract and may reinfect at a later stage. However, new antiviral drugs are being developed which may soon enable a chemotherapeutic approach to treating the virus.

If I have had my cervical pre-cancer treated and I develop it again, what sort of treatment should I have?
Treatment depends on the results and recommendations of repeated investigations of cervical smear, colposcopy, and biopsy as for your initial disease.

How many times can I be re-treated?
As many times as is required.

What are the dangers/drawbacks of re-treatment of pre-cancer?

There are no specific dangers associated with re-treatment for cervical pre-cancer. The potential drawbacks include further loss of cervical tissue, which if repeated, may diminish the volume of cervix to an extent where it may become less 'competent', particularly if the treatment involves a cone biopsy. This can cause problems supporting a pregnancy, but can be overcome by inserting a stitch into the cervix. There may also be a problem with inadequate dilation of the cervix at the time of delivery, which can necessitate delivery by Caesarean section.

I have had an abnormal smear and at colposcopic examination the consultant told me I have a pre-cancer which will need treatment. Reading the list of risk factors, I don't consider myself as having run any of these. I have never smoked, I have not been promiscuous, I have one husband, who works as a miner. He denies being promiscuous, so how could I have got this disease? How long have I had it, as my previous smear taken only three years ago, was normal? I have only had one child, and I don't see how I could have got this infection.

It is possible for you to have become affected even if you have had only one sexual partner. Prior to meeting you, he may have had sex with someone who had a viral infection without knowing it, and he may be an unwitting and silent carrier of an agent responsible for inducing the disease. Your husband's job as a miner is recognized as being a high risk factor in cervical cancer. It may be that some aspect of his work renders his semen more likely to cause changes to the cervix which subsequently becomes pre-cancerous. He may also have some of the risk factors outlined in a previous chapter which may make him more likely to induce abnormalities in your cervical skin. The previous normal smear taken three years ago may not have shown any abnormality, either because none had developed at that time, or, more rarely, because the smear sampling may have failed to scrape and pick up abnormal cells despite the fact that they existed on the cervix.

How long should I wait after biopsy, local ablative treatment, cone biopsy or a hysterectomy before resuming sexual intercourse?

If a biopsy is taken, sexual intercourse should be avoided for one week to allow the tissue to heal. Following local ablative treatment, intercourse should be avoided for up to six weeks. After cone biopsy, which is a more drastic type of surgery, the interval may be longer, depending on how much tissue has been removed and low long the remaining tissue takes to heal. Following a hysterectomy, intercourse should be avoided until the all-clear from a doctor, which is usually six weeks to two months after the operation.

What is an erosion and does it have anything to do with cervical cancer?

An erosion is an area of skin on the cervix covered by a lining which originally came from inside the cervical canal. These cells are still undergoing some changes from columnar to squamous epithelium. This area on the transformation zone has a tendency to bleed, get infected and is a prime site on which pre-cancerous changes can take place. If bleeding or infection is recurrent and troublesome, the 'eroded' transformation zone can be destroyed by one of the local treatments used for treating pre-cancer. The treatment most frequently used is cryosurgery (freezing). Before such destruction, it is vital to check for CIN to ensure that the proposed type of treatment and depth of destruction is correctly carried out. If CIN is present, it may have to be treated in a different way. Occasionally, a new 'erosion' can occur some time after treatment. The erosion itself does not cause the development of pre-cancer but happens to be the site at which pre-cancer can occur. Taking the Pill can increase the likelihood of occurence of erosion, particularly at an early age, when the Pill increases the surface area of the transformation zone on which pre-cancerous changes can take place.

If the cervical smear reported does not contain endocervical cells, should it be regarded as unsatisfactory?

Ideally, a smear should contain cells from all areas of the cervix, including the cervical canal. If endocervical cells are missing, the cytologist is not in a position to know whether or not an abnormality exists in the endocervical canal. If the smear is otherwise normal, a repeat smear should be performed in the near future (e.g. a year later) to include endocervical cells, in order to confirm that the endocervical canal has been sampled. This is most important in post-menopausal women in whom the disease may hide in the endocervical canal.

What is a local ablative treatment?
Treatment aimed at removing all the diseased skin from the cervix.

What is the difference between local ablative treatment and a cone biopsy?
With the exception of diathermy loop excision, local ablative treatment destroys diseased tissue from an abnormal area which has been seen and identified in its entirety. With the exception of diathermy, such treatments can be carried out on an out-patient basis and the removal of the tissue is therefore performed by one of the physical methods of burning or freezing. No tissue is available at a later stage for re-examination as the whole diseased area has been destroyed. Cone biopsy, in contrast, is a diagnostic technique that involves cutting out the abnormal area from the cervix and the tissue in its entirety is saved for histological assessment and future re-examination. Cone biopsy involves a greater amount of tissue being removed and, until recently, had to be done on an in-patient basis and without colposcopy, resulting in greater damage to the cervix. Using colposcopy and cutting out the tissue using a laser or knife it has been possible to reduce the risks involved with cone biopsy. In some centres, this technique has recently become an out-patient procedure with local rather than general anaesthetic.

Will local ablative treatment cure me, or will the pre-cancer reoccur?
When such treatment is advised by the colposcopist, the chances of a complete cure after one treatment are very high (93 per cent). The other 7 per cent need further treatment. The earlier one catches the abnormality the greater the likelihood of complete eradication and prevention of progression towards invasive cancer. However, once treated, it is possible for the disease to re-occur as a result of some residual pre-cancerous cells, or occur anew. Therefore regular follow-up examinations including a smear, with or without colposcopy, are necessary at intervals suggested by the gynaecologist or laboratory. The more severe and widespread

the original disease, the more likely it is to re-occur. It is less likely to re-occur when a large and deep area is removed from the cervix because this is a better guarantee that the disease has been completely removed. The larger the abnormal area on the transformation zone, the more likely a disease is to re-occur.

I have had a complete hysterectomy. Do I need cervical smears after that, as the cervix will no longer be there?
If the hysterectomy was carried out for non-malignant reasons, such as uterine fibroids, then smears from the vagina and vaginal vault should still be taken at three to five yearly intervals. There may still exist a very remote chance of a pre-cancer in that area even after hysterectomy. However, if the hysterectomy was performed because of cervical pre-cancer, cancer or other malignancy, then annual smears need to be carried out with additional colposcopy to detect or exclude a likelihood of any residual or new abnormality.

What protection does the cap give?
It provides a better barrier than the Pill or IUD against potential effects of semen on the cervix, but is not quite as good as the condom, because semen (which may carry cancer-inducing agents) is still deposited in the vagina.

What protection does a condom give?
British Standard-tested condoms should prevent transmission of bacteria and viruses present on and in the penis. They also prevent the transmission of semen, which may contain agents involved in inducing cervical cancer.

How reliable is a post-menopausal cervical smear?
It is likely to be reliable if it includes cells from all the areas of the cervix, including endocervical cells. In post-menopausal women, the transformation zone has been drawn up into the endocervical canal which subsequently narrows with age. Sampling the potentially suspect area is difficult, and a specialized spatula capable of reaching and sampling this area should be used to help retrieve endocervical cells, as well as sampling the entire cervical area. Taking smears at a maximum interval of three years should increase the reliability of detection of abnormal cells.

When can a post-menopausal woman stop having smears?
Generally smears may stop after a woman is 65 if she has not had sexual intercourse for three years. However, if a woman did not have a smear in her 60s, an undetected pre-cancer may manifest itself many years later and a cancer appearing in a woman's seventies or eighties may be a reflection of a disease which began many years earlier. Therefore, elderly women who did not have smears for more than three years before their 70th birthday should have a smear. Smears may cease after this age if there have been three successive negative smears and no further intercourse.

At what age am I free from cervical cancer?
Women have been known to have cervical cancer in their eighties, often presenting as an invasive, widely disseminating disease. These women usually had not had a cervical smear for years, or not at all.

Does the use of vaginal tampons increase the risk of cervical cancer?
So far, statistics have shown that this is unlikely.

Can vaginal tampons be used after treatment?
They should be avoided for around two months after treatment to prevent the cervix being rubbed and chafed by the tampon and to allow the treated areas on the cervix to heal properly.

Is the IUD linked to cervical cancer?
There is no evidence that an IUD in itself causes cervical cancer, but, because it leaves the cervix exposed to contact with semen, there is therefore a greater risk of exposure to some form of sexually transmitted disease, such as cervical cancer, than if a condom or cap were used.

Does an IUD have to be removed prior to local ablative treatment?
You can sometimes have treatment with the IUD in place, but the strings occasionally get in the way of treatment and so the IUD may need to be removed at the time of treatment and a new one inserted afterwards.

Is it safe to have a smear and/or colposcopy during pregnancy?
Yes.

Is it safe to have a biopsy during pregnancy?
Biopsy is usually avoided during pregnancy unless the smear and colposcopy suggests the presence of an advanced pre-cancer or cancer. In this case, a wedge biopsy, a crescent shaped small piece of tissue may be removed. There is no major danger of miscarriage as a result of this procedure.

Is it safe to have a cone biopsy during pregnancy?
There is a significant risk of miscarriage which is greater if the cone biopsy is performed in the later stages of pregnancy (four months onwards).

I have recently had an abnormal smear, in fact severe dyskaryosis had been diagnosed. I want to have a baby so I went to have another smear and this smear was normal. I was told I could go ahead and try for a baby. I have not had a colposcopic examination. What should I do?
You would be very unwise to rely on a normal smear which has followed a severely dyskaryotic smear, and colposcopy should be performed, and another smear taken under colposcopic examination so that an all-clear verdict is given before you attempt to have the baby.

I am pregnant and have had an abnormal smear. What happens next?
You should be advised by your gynaecologist and cytologist about the type of follow-up. If they recommend colposcopy then this needs to be carried out by a specialist who knows how to interpret findings in pregnancy as an abnormality on the cervix in pregnancy may be difficult to understand and interpret. Colposcopy will identify the presence and extent of abnormal areas. Biopsies are avoided as far as possible. It is necessary to repeat colposcopic surveillance during pregnancy to ensure that the disease is not progressing and if there is a slightest suspicion of this, a special wedge biopsy needs to be taken to exclude invasion.

Most abnormal smears in pregnancy can be followed up in this manner. Colposcopic examination and smear is essential six to ten weeks after the delivery and if the abnormality persists, then it should be treated in the usual way.

Will cervical cancer affect my pregnancy?
If the disease is only in the pre-cancerous state, and is carefully

monitored under expert colposcopic surveillance to ensure that it is not invasive, treatment can be delayed until after the delivery, if the disease persists. Its presence should not affect the ability of the cervix to function normally during pregnancy and delivery. The only time the pregnancy is likely to be affected is when the examinations have shown that the disease has become invasive and major operative procedures are needed, either to prevent it from spreading or to save the life of the mother. Such procedures may result in aborting the foetus or in its early delivery. This is a rare occurrence in countries where women are likely to be screened well before the disease has reached an invasive stage.

Will treatment affect my chances of having a baby?
Local treatments, especially laser treatment, are not likely to affect the chances of becoming pregnant or carrying and delivering a baby. If a cone biopsy is needed, this may affect the chances of carrying the pregnancy to term and delivering the baby vaginally. It all depends on the amount of tissue removed and subsequent damage to the cervix by the cone biopsy.

Is it all right to conceive while waiting for pre-cancer treatment?
It is best to wait until after treatment. Treatment will remove diseased skin from the cervix and remove the worry during pregnancy that the pre-cancer may progress or become invasive.

Does genital herpes carry an increased risk of cervical cancer?
For many years it was suspected that genital herpes was associated with or had a role to play in causing cervical cancer. However, recent work carried out now suggests this is unlikely.

Can promiscuity be blamed for cervical pre-cancer or cancer?
A lot of evidence seems to suggest that cervical cancer is a sexually transmitted disease. With increased number of partners there is an increased chance of acquiring it and possibly transmitting an agent which induces the disease in other people. Among the sexually transmitted infections, the human papilloma virus seems to be the chief contender suspected of taking part in inducing pre-cancerous changes, however, there may be other infections which have a role to play in cervical cancer, but which are yet to be identified.

Does circumcision reduce the risk of transmitting HPV?

Circumcision will not reduce the risk of transmitting any infective organism such as HPV. However, it may make identification of penile warts easier as they often grow under the foreskin, which is removed during circumcision.

I keep having to have repeat smears and each time they find some abnormal cells. How long will this go on for and why do I keep on having repeat smears?

Not all abnormal cells are or will become cancerous. Your cervical smears have probably shown an abnormality which may not appear to be pre-cancerous. For reasons such as the presence of a vaginal discharge causing an obscured smear, an infection, or inflammation, it may not be possible to fully assess the state of the cervical cells as regards cancerous change. Therefore if an abnormality persists then the smear should be repeated, preferably under colposcopic surveillance and a biopsy taken to identify the nature and extent of any abnormality seen.

What happens if my pre-cancer is not treated?

While mild pre-cancer may, in some cases, regress to normal, it is not possible to distinguish at present which will regress and which will progress to cancer. Along with moderate and severe forms the pre-cancer can become invasive and eventually invade into the cervix and then metastasize (spread) beyond the reach of effective treatment. At present, it is not possible to predict if, how, and when this may happen, as it is a very individual thing. By removing abnormal cells in their pre-cancerous state, such progression should be stopped.

Who are the women at risk of acquiring cervical cancer?

Every woman is at risk of cervical cancer, particularly those who have been or are sexually active. But the women at the greatest risk are those who do not present themselves for smears.

Why is it that there has been such an increase in the numbers of young women being affected by this disease?

There is no definite and easy answer. Women have taken to smoking and this has been shown to be one of the major risk factors involved in causing cancer, including cervical cancer. The Pill has liberated women from the fear of pregnancy and has resulted in fewer barrier methods of contraception (such as condom or cap) being used. This has made it easier for women to become infected by organisms or other agents transmitted by their partners. With more women being infected and having more sexual partners, more men may become infected and in turn infect more women — a snowball effect.

There is increasing evidence that inflammation caused by infective organisms may in some way facilitate the onset of cervical cancer. Whether this is by direct action or by paving the way for another infective agent is not known.

There also seems to have been a change in recent years in the nature of the disease. It seems to have become more aggressive, especially so in younger women under 35 years of age and proceeds to more advanced stages more quickly than before.

Chapter 16

Winning the battle

MODERN TREATMENT of cervical pre-cancer involves diagnosing it in its earliest possible form and arranging for its complete removal before it spreads and affects other organs in the body. Fortunately, cervical cancer begins as a localized *in situ* pre-cancer, which means there is a chance of eradicating it before it develops into an invasive cancer which is much harder to treat and presents a threat to fertility, and ultimately to a woman's life. The problem is that we do not know what causes the disease. Several predisposing factors have been identified as being implicated in the development and progression of cervical cancer. We thought at one time that we did have an idea of the time scale of development and progression. This is why, many years ago the government recommendation was that women should be screened at five-yearly intervals. This was thought to be following the natural pattern of the disease and there was no need to screen more often. The new guidelines of a smear every three years reflect recent evidence which has clearly shown that cervical cancer can, in some cases, progress very quickly from being a mild cervical abnormality to a cancerous one. Although the disease usually takes many years to progress there also seems to be a more aggressive form which can progress to CIN 3 or even further within a year on rare occasions.

In an ideal world, we would suggest that all women should have a smear every year from the onset of intercourse, to the age of 70. This would not only take account of the possible rapid progression of the disease, but would also reduce the risk of the effects of receiving a falsely reassuring negative result.

The financial implications of implementing a screening programme of this magnitude precludes it from becoming a reality in the near future. More realistic, and almost as effective, is to ensure that every woman has a smear at least every three years and that those who have had abnormal smears are smeared annually. This should really be a right rather than a privilege. However, even this is a far more radical and expensive approach than suggested by most governments, even in the West.

Some would regard this as 'over-screening', and in the past this may have been true, but it is now becoming apparent that cervical pre-cancers are developing faster than ever before, and screening guidelines based on old statistics do not give the true picture witnessed by those working in the field of cervical cancer.

One of the reasons women do not have regular smears is that they are not aware of their importance. Between 60 and 90 per cent of women who die of cervical cancer have never had a smear. Some of the reasons for this were examined in an earlier chapter and we would emphasize the need for advertising and information campaigns to bring the message home that smears are an effective means of detecting cervical cancer at a pre-cancerous and treatable stage. Such a campaign should educate women that a treatable pre-cancerous condition exists. Many women do not want a smear because they think a positive result will mean that they have a cancer for which little can be done. It would also help to have literature available in libraries and doctor's surgeries, or inserted as leaflets in women's periodicals.

One new organization, Women Against Cervical Cancer (WACC), has recently started to beat the drum for more screening services. It was started by Annabel Cutter who was rightly angered that more than 2,000 women are dying from the disease each year in Britain. Perhaps if the call for a better screening system became louder, it would become more of a political issue with votes at stake and money may become available. While it costs a lot of money to run the type of screening system we have suggested above, by preventing the onset of invasive cancer, thousands of pounds per patient can be saved in terms of long-term hospital stay, expensive treatment, and the loss to the Exchequer of income tax from their earnings. The most important saving is the cost of a life to women and their families.

On the positive side, the number of smears being taken has gone up by around 50 per cent in the last ten years. Progress has been made, particularly when one considers that in the same time the number of positive smears detected has trebled. This suggests that the prevalence of the disease is increasing so more facilities are needed to provide colposcopy and enable conservative local treatment to be carried out.

At present, colposcopy is almost exclusively a hospital-based service, but there is no reason why it should not become a GP-based one. It would need government help, as GPs would be understandably reluctant to invest many thousands of pounds in buying the equipment. One possible way is for GPs to be paid a fee for colposcopy, as they are for taking smears. If the Government is serious about preventive medicine then we suggest that this is one avenue they should consider, particularly as it would free hospital consultants from time-consuming colposcopy.

As regards the future, there are many researchers looking at what causes the cancer to develop in the first place. We have mentioned various predisposing factors which may facilitate the onset of cervical abnormalities. In the last couple of years, US researchers have become further convinced that there is overwhelming evidence linking the wart virus, particularly the type HPV 16, to cervical cancer, while the British doctors are not all quite so convinced. New techniques involving DNA hybridization and polymerase chain reactions have enabled rapid detection of HPV and other infections in cervical samples. Using these techniques, screening large numbers of patients will enable researchers to correlate the presence of HPV and other infective agents with the onset of cervical abnormalities.

However, on the basis that HPV is implicated in some way, Dr Lionel Crawford, head of the Imperial Research Fund's tumour virus group at Cambridge, announced in September 1990 that steps towards a vaccine were underway. Genes taken from HPV 16 had been incorporated into another virus which when injected into animals had caused a protective antibody response. Researchers hope to develop the technique to use as a vaccine in humans whereby the body's immune system would be enhanced to destroy the virus. Though Dr Crawford suggested that such a vaccine was years away he was 'very optimistic' that, following animal tests, it was the first step towards a vaccine.

Once such a vaccine is developed, it could be given in two ways: to children, both boys and girls, to give general protection in the community against the virus; and as a form of therapy for women to prevent pre-malignant cells in cervical tissue from turning cancerous.

Ironically, the emergence of the AIDS epidemic and the subsequent increase in the promotion and use of condoms, may have a beneficial effect in protecting women from viral transmission.

Another area of interest as regards the cause of cervical abnormality is the role of hormones in cervical cancer, in that they may have a possible part to play, much in the same way as they have been implicated in breast cancer. If such links were to be found then it may be possible to develop blood tests for these as early diagnostic signs and it may then be possible to tailor specific drugs which may prevent the induction of cancer.

By being so accessible for investigations, the cervix provides an excellent site for research into cancer. It is possible that this research will provide understanding of other types of cancer.

What is needed now?

Resources are now needed to finance a veritable army of researchers from all branches of science, to join forces in the battle against cervical cancer. This battle will only be won when we can save all those women destined to die from it, and prevent the disease completely.

Until this happens we would hope that any woman reading this book will take home the message that at present our chief weapon against this disease is the cervical smear, and that the aim of cervical screening is to detect pre-cancer which if caught early can be treated, often with up to 100 per cent chance of a complete cure. Hopefully any male readers will encourage their female partners, friends and relatives to have a regular smear.

Glossary of terms

Acetic acid   Pure vinegar, usually used in a dilute form as a diagnostic dye to identify abnormal areas on the cervix.

Aceto-white areas   Suspected areas of abnormality as indicated by their white appearance following acetic acid application.

Actinomycetes   A fungus, often found in vaginal and uterine fluids, occurring in association with intrauterine coil devices (IUD) except when devices include copper.

Adenocarcinoma (of the cervix)   Cancer arising in the glands of the columnar cervical epithelium situated in the cervical canal.

AIDS (Acquired immune deficiency syndrome)   Destruction of body defences by their invasion with the virus called human immunodeficiency virus.

Anaerobes   Organisms, such as bacteria or fungi, which can live without oxygen.

Anaerobic bacteria   Bacteria which live without oxygen and may be found in moist airless genital tracts.

Anucleates   Cells without a nucleus.

Atrophy/atrophic   Shrinking.

Atypia   Deviating from normal appearance.

Atypical squamous metaplasia   See *Metaplasia*.

Auto-immune disease   A defence reaction by the body's immune system to one's own tissue (a self-destructive phenomenon).

Aylesbury spatula   A new version of the Ayres spatula, with a narrow wooden prong suitable for sampling the endocervical canal.

Ayres spatula   Type of wooden spatula used in taking cervical smears.

Bacteria   Microscopic organisms capable of infecting tissues.

Basement membrane   The tissue barrier separating the cervical skin from the underlying deeper tissues containing blood vessels and lymphatic channels.

Biopsy   A sample piece of tissue removed for laboratory examination by punching it out with biopsy forceps (punch biopsy) or cutting out a thin wedge (wedge biopsy) or by using a hot wire (loop biopsy).

Caesarean section   Incision through the abdomen and then the uterus to remove the foetus. This procedure is performed when normal vaginal delivery is contraindicated or impossible.

Cancer   Where cells undergo a change within them and acquire an unlimited and uncontrolled growth. They grow into, penetrate, and invade the surrounding underlying tissues, forming malignant tumours (abnormal masses of cancerous cells). Such cells may break off and spread (metastasis) via the lymphatic channels and the blood stream to other organs where they may lodge and similarly multiply uncontrollably into tumours.

Candida   Fungi, also known as Monilia or thrush, often flourishing in the female genital tracts and also in the mouths of infants. Often lives in the rectum, but can be transferred to the genital tract where it causes itching, irritation, and discharge.

Carcinogen   Any substance capable of causing normal tissues to become cancerous.

Carcinoma   A medical term synonymous with cancer but not used to describe cancer of muscle or bone (sarcoma).

Carcinoma in situ   The point at which pre-cancerous cells have become cancerous but are still confined to the cervical skin.

Cautery/cauterization   Physical destruction of an area of affected cervical skin with subsequent coagulation of underlying bleeding vessels. This can be via freezing (cryocautery or cyotherapy) or burning (diathermy).

Cell   Basic unit from which tissue is built. Most have a nucleus which contains the genetic material (DNA), and this is surrounded by cytoplasm which in turn is surrounded by a cell membrane which separates it from other adjoining cells.

Cervical intraepithelial neoplasia (CIN)   This describes the state of precancerous abnormality confined to the cervical skin as indicated by a biopsy (removal of piece of tissue which is subsequently analysed in the laboratory). The degree of abnormality is denoted by suffixing the abreviation CIN with number 1, 2, or 3, the latter being the most severe and least likely to revert to normal.

Cervicography   A technique for taking photographs of the cervix after it has been stained with acetic acid, for the purpose of identification of abnormal areas on the cervix or to make a permanent pictorial record of the state of the cervix. Such photographs can be taken by personnel not trained in colposcopy, thus freeing colposcopists to concentrate on interpretation of results from photographs. The technique can also be used to follow the progression of the disease by comparing photographs of mild abnormalities with photographs taken later on.

Cervix   The neck of the uterus (womb).

Chemotherapy   Treatment using drugs.

Chlamydia   Minute parasitic organisms which live inside the cells of the genital tract and may cause pelvic inflammatory disease which may result in blocked Fallopian tubes. They can also live in conjunctivae (eyelid lining) of the eyes and cause a discharge from the site.

CIN   See *Cervical intraepithelial neoplasia.*

Cold coagulation   Heat destruction of an abnormal area of the cervix but referred to as being 'cold' because the technique employs a probe at 100°C as opposed to up to 1000°C used in diathermy.

Colposcope   Low-powered binocular microscope with a light source which allows for inspection of the surface of the vagina and cervix.

Colposcopy   The use of a colposcope to identify the presence, extent, and type of abnormality of the cervix.

Columnar cells   Column-shaped cells found in columnar epithelium which lines the endocervical canal.

Columnar epithelium   Lining containing columnar cells, such as is found in the endocervical canal. This lining is a single cell layer thick and is responsible for producing mucus. It is situated mainly in the cervical canal leading from the vagina to the uterus.

Condom   Rubberized protective cover placed over the penis before sexual intercourse to prevent sperm entering the vagina or cervix, thus preventing fertilization of an egg and hence the onset of pregnancy. Condoms are also used to prevent the transfer of infective agents during sexual intercourse.

Cone biopsy   Removal of a cone-shaped piece of tissue from the cervix using a knife or laser. This is performed when a cervical abnormality is suspected as a result of cytology and its full extent cannot be determined by colposcopy or ordinary small biopsies, or where colposcopy facilities are unavailable.

Cryocautery (cryotherapy)   Local treatment often used to treat cervical pre-cancer which involves inserting a probe into the cervix, and freezing the diseased tissue using carbon dioxide or nitrous oxide.

Curettage   Use of a special long-handled metal scraper to scrape the lining of the uterus in order to check whether the cells of the uterine lining are normal.

Cytobrush   Long thin implement like a pipe-cleaner, used to sample cells from the cervical canal in order to take a cervical smear.

Cytology   Study of cells.

Cytometry   The counting and measuring of cells.

Cytoplasm   Contents of the cell excluding the nucleus.

Diathermy (electrocoagulation)   Electrically generated heat (up to 1000°C) used to burn off pre-cancerous abnormalities on the cervix.

Dilatation and curettage (D and C)   This is where the cervical canal has been distended or widened (dilatation) to enable cells to be scraped from the canal or uterus using a scoop or spoon (curettage) in order to examine cells under the microscope to check for abnormalities. D and C is performed when abnormalities detected on a smear suggest the presence of uterine abnormalities.

DNA (Deoxyribonucleic acid)   This is the molecule within the nucleus of cells which carries the genetic code and dictates tissue development.

Dyskaryosis/dyskaryotic (dys = bad, karyosis = nucleus)   The nuclear abnormality of the cells observed on a cervical smear, and the degree of such disturbance is described as mild, moderate, or severe dyskaryosis.

Dysplasia (dys = bad, plasia = formation) Malformation of cells and tissues. Originally used as a histological and cytological term to describe such abnormalities. It has now been replaced as a cytological term (i.e. in describing smears) by 'dyskaryosis' which is a more specific description of nuclear abnormality within cells. 'Dysplasia' is still used by some centres internationally, although it should now only be used in a histological assessment of a biopsy.

Ectocervix The vaginal area of the cervix.

Ectropion The correct medical term for an erosion.

Endocervical canal This is the canal which leads from the cervical opening to the main body of the uterus.

Endocervical cells Cells from the endocervical canal.

Endocervical curettage Scraping away the lining of the cervical canal. The lining is examined under the microscope for the presence of adenocarcinoma or squamous cell carcinoma.

Endocervical epithelium The epithelium lining the endocervical canal. It contains columnar cells, so named because of their columnar shape.

Endocervical glands Mucus-producing glands which line the endocervical canal.

Endometrium Mucus membrane lining the uterus. It is this lining which breaks down in the absence of fertilization of the egg by sperm, and is released during menstruation.

Epithelium Technical term for skin.

Erosion A reddened and raised area of columnar epithelium around the external cervical os.

Excision Cut out.

Exenteration Extensive surgical removal of organs within the pelvis. This is performed in cases of persistent invasive cancer which is not eradicated by more conservative treatment.

Exfoliate Medical term for flake or peel off.

False negative A result, such as from a smear or colposcopic investigation, which mistakenly indicates that all is well where in fact an abnormality exists.

False positive   A smear or colposcopy result which suggests existence of an abnormality where in fact there is no abnormality.

Gamma rays   The form of radiation used in radiotherapy. It is used in treating invasive cervical cancer.

General Practitioner (GP)   Family doctor concerned with general health of patients.

Genital tract   Includes all structures relating or belonging to reproduction.

Genital warts   A skin growth of variable size which may be round, flat, soft or hard, and occurs in response to papilloma virus infection.

Glandular epithelium   Skin which contains glands.

Glandular neoplasia   Cancer of cervical glands, i.e. adenocarcinoma or cancer in uterine endometrium.

Glycogen   A form of sugar stored in human tissues.

High vaginal swab (HVS)   A sample of vaginal discharge obtained from the endocervical and vaginal canal taken in cases of vaginal discharge to identify the presence of bacteria and fungi. This should not be confused with a cervical smear.

Histology/histologist/histopathologist   Histology is the study of the structure of tissues. A histologist studies normal tissues whereas a histopathologist is concerned with indentifying abnormalities in diseased tissues.

Hormone   A chemical substance usually produced by glands which is carried by ducts or the bloodstream to another part of the body where it exerts an effect.

Human papilloma virus (HPV)   See *Wart virus*.

Hysterectomy   Removal of the uterus. (This term does not really describe all the tissues that may be removed at such an operation, e.g. uterus, including cervix; uterus with one or both Fallopian tubes and ovaries). See also *Wertheim's Hysterectomy*.

Immunology   Branch of science concerned with immunity to disease.

Inflammation   Redness, heat, swelling and pain which occurs when tissue responds to physical or chemical injury or infection by an organism. This results from the arrival in the infected area of lymphocytes (often called inflammatory cells) and other white cells such as monocytes and polymorphonuclear leucocytes.

Invasive cancer   Cancer cells invading blood and lymph channels.

Koilocytes   Cells in which the nucleus appears to be surrounded by halo, usually in response to a viral infection often by human papilloma virus.

Langerhans cells   Cells found in the pancreas which are responsible for production of insulin, or cells found under the surface of the skin including the cervix thought to be concerned with presenting carcinogens to the lymphocytes which are able to recognize and often to neutralize them.

Laser   The laser beam is a form of high intensity light energy which is capable of cutting out or vaporizing abnormal cervical tissue causing minimal damage to surrounding tissues.

Local ablative treatment (LAT)   Local removal of diseased tissues.

Loop biopsy/excision   (also known as DLE — diathermy loop excision, or LLETZ — large loop excision of the transformation zone). A recently introduced diagnostic and treatment technique where an electrically-heated wire loop is used to remove the transformation zone.

Lymph glands   Equivalent to lymph nodes. These are small nodules of lymphatic tissues situated along the lymph channels into which lymph from tissues drain. They also produce lymphocytes.

Lymphatic channels   Thin-walled vessels which conduct and drain excess tissue fluid into the blood stream.

Lymphocytes   White blood cells produced by lymph glands, spleen and bone marrow; part of in the body's defences against infection.

Malignant   Describes cells capable of uncontrolled multiplication, growth and spread to other tissues with a subsequent capability of killing the host.

Menopause   The time when there are a number of hormonal changes, of which cessation of menstruation is just one of the many manifestations which can be sudden or of a gradually diminishing nature. The menopause usually occurs in a woman's

194

late 40s or 50s, and is sometimes referred to as 'the change'.

Menstruation   Hormonally-controlled shedding of the uterine lining which subsequently passes out as a bloody discharge from the vagina. Occurs at regular cyclical intervals, usually every 28 days although in some women the cycles may be regularly shorter or longer or even completely irregular.

Metaplasia (meta = half, plasia = formation)   A normal, non-malignant replacement of one type of tissue by another, e.g. columnar epithelium replaced by squamous epithelium on the transformation zone. Atypical metaplasia—when metaplastic cells appear atypical. Immature metaplasia—this is when squamous metaplasia is not yet complete. Squamous metaplasia—substitution of columnar epithelium by squamous epithelium.

Metastasis   Transfer of cancerous cells to other parts of the body via the lymphatics, blood channels, or by direct contact.

Microinvasive carcinoma   Describes the situation where cells with a highly cancerous potential have broken through the basement membrane which separates the cervical skin from underlying deeper structures, to a depth not greater than three millimetres.

Monilia   See *Candida*.

Neoplasia (neo = new, plasia = formation)   Growth of new abnormal tissue which may become cancerous.

Normal smear   Adequate sample of cells from the cervix which contains normal cells only.

Nucleus   The part of a cell which contains the genetic material (DNA) and is surrounded by a nuclear membrane and cytoplasm.

Os   External: The opening or mouth in the cervix which leads into the cervical canal. Internal: The opening at the top of the cervical canal leading into the uterus.

Palliative treatment   Treatment which alleviates pain and the severity of a disease, but is not a cure.

Pap smear   Same as a cervical smear.

Papanicolaou, George Nicholas (1889-1962)   Developer of the Pap smear test for diagnosing cervical cancer, and now also pre-cancer. The Pap test is nowadays referred to as the smear test.

Pre-cancer The situation when tissues have changed from normal and are at a stage where they have a potential to become cancerous. Such changes are described as cervical intrapithelial neoplasia (CIN), the degree of abnormality being defined as CIN 1, CIN 2 or CIN 3, as the severity increases. Pre-cancers are confined to the tissue in which they arose and once they acquire potential spread beyond it, they cease to be pre-cancers.

Radiotherapy Treatment using radiation.
Rectum The back passage.

Semen Fluid produced by the prostate gland and the testes, the latter producing the sperm which are responsible for fertilization.
Spatula Plastic or wooden stick used to take a cervical smear.
Speculum An instrument used to open the vagina to enable the taking of a smear, or colposcopy.
Squamocolumnar junction The meeting point of the columnar epithelium of the endocervical canal and the squamous epithelium of the vagina.
Squamous cell carcinoma A cancer occurring in the squamous epithelium.
Squamous epithelium A sheet of multi-layered cells which line, among other parts of the body, the vagina and part of the cervix.
Squamous metaplasia Substitution of columnar epithelium by squamous epithelium.
Staging Description of the spread of cancer. The higher the stage, the more invasive the cancer.
Stenosis A medical term describing tightening or narrowing. The cervical canal of post-menopausal women is often 'stenosed'.

Thrush See *Candida*.
Transformation zone (TZ) The area on the cervix which is covered by the migrated columnar epithelium from the cervical canal. It is the area which undergoes squamous metaplasia and it is also the prime site where cervical pre-cancer is thought to begin.
Trichomonas A sexually transmitted type of protozoa found in the vagina. The infection with Trichomonas may cause inflammation and bad smelling vaginal discharge.

Tumour   A growth or swelling. If a tumour is benign, its growth is limited to one particular area. If the tumour is malignant (i.e. cancerous) it has the potential for spread to other parts of the body and may ultimately prove fatal.

Uterus (the womb)   A muscular thick-walled structure surrounding a cavity. Its lining is known as the endometrium and it is here that a fertilized egg implant develops into a baby. If fertilization does not occur, the lining is shed in menstruation.

Vagina   The canal which extends from the cervix to an external opening between the labia minora (the vaginal lips).

Vault smears   Vaginal smears from women who have had a hysterectomy.

Virus   A tiny micro-organism, much smaller than a bacteria, whose presence can be detected under an electron microscope. Viruses cause damage by releasing their genetic material into human cells in which they subsequently replicate, causing such cells to burst open, releasing large numbers of viral particles. Some are implicated in causing cancer of various organs.

Wart virus   Term commonly used to describe the human papilloma virus, several types of which have been implicated as the agent transmitted during sexual intercourse which induces cervical cancer. This virus can cause warts to grow on the penis, vulva, vagina, rectum, and elsewhere. It may also exist in these tissues without visible warts. There is evidence that it may be transmitted during sexual intercourse. Part of the viral protein of certain types of the wart virus have been found to form a new cancer protein in the cancer cells of the cervix.

Wedge biopsy   Thin slice of tissue removed by knife or laser. Performed when cone biopsy may be dangerous, such as in pregnancy.

Wertheim's Hysterectomy   A hysterectomy which removes the uterus and its appendages, including the Fallopian tubes, ligaments, and ovaries. It also removes pelvic lymph nodes and any other nodes which are suspected of containing malignant cells.

Appendix

Printed in the UK for HMSO. D.8194398 2,000m 10/89. 36625.

WRITE CLEARLY WITH BALLPOINT PEN ON A HARD SURFACE OR BACK COPY WILL BE ILLEGIBLE

ENTER DETAILS IN BOXES OR RING APPROPRIATE NUMBERS

Fold for B

Fold for A

FORM HMR 101/5 (1989) Multi-copy

01 Woman's hospital registration number

02 Laboratory

03 Woman's surname _____ Previous surname _____

First names _____

Full postal address _____

_____ post code _____

04 Date of birth _____ / _____ / _____   **05 NHS number** _____

06 If hospital state consultant, clinic or ward, and hospital

A Name and address of sender if not GP

_____ post code _____

07 **B** Name and address of GP

_____ post code _____

08 GP's FPC code

09 Source of smear		10
GP _____ 1	NHS hospital _____ 4	LOCAL __
NHS community clinic __ 2	Private _____ 5	
GUM clinic _____ 3	Other _____ 6	CODES __

Request/report for cervical or vaginal cytology – GP's COPY

198

11 Code number of laboratory	*Fold*	12 Slide serial number

CLINICAL REPORT

Date of:

13 this test ____ / ____ / ____

14 LMP (1st day) ____ / ____ / ____

15 last test ____ / ____ / ____

16 If no previous test please put X [ ]

17 Reason for smear

routine call _____ 1

routine recall _____ 2

clinically indicated _____ 3

previous abnormal smear _____ 4

18 Specimen type

cervical scrape _____ 1

other (specify) _____ 2

19 Condition

pregnant _____ 1

post-natal (under 12 weeks) _____ 2

I.U.C.D. fitted _____ 3

taking hormones (specify in 20) _____ 4

20 Clinical data (including signs and symptoms, previous abnormal cytology with slide number, previous diagnosis and treatment)

signature

21 CYTOLOGY REPORT

22 Cytological pattern		23 Specific infection		24 Management suggested	
inadequate specimen	1	trichomonas	1	normal recall	1
negative	2	candida	2	repeat smear	
borderline changes	8	wart virus	3	in ___ months	2
mild dyskaryosis	3	herpes	4	or after treatment	3
moderate dyskaryosis	7	actinomyces	5	gynaecological referral	4
severe dyskaryosis	4	other (specify)	6	cancel recall	5
severe dyskaryosis/ ? invasive carcinoma	5	**Signature**		date	
? glandular neoplasia	6				

_1 _4

_2 _5

_3 _6

Centres for advice and counselling

UK
British Association of Cancer United Patients
121-123 Charterhouse Street
London EC1M 6AA
Tel: 071 608 1661
Freephone 0800 181199

BUPA Women's Unit
300 Gray's Inn Road
London WC1
Tel: 071 837 6484

Cancerlink
17 Britannia Street
London WC1X 9JN
Tel: 071 833 2451

The Family Planning Association
27-35 Mortimer Street
London W1N 7JR
Tel: 071 636 7866

Hysterectomy Support Groups
11 Henryson Road
London SE4 1HL
Tel: 081 690 5987

Marie Stopes House
108 Whitfield Street
London W1
Tel: 071 388 0662/2585

Women's Health Concern
83 Earls Court Road
London W8
Tel: 081 938 3932

Women's Health Information Centre
52 Featherstone Street
London EC1 8RT
Tel: 071 251 6580

Women's National Cancer Control Campaign
1 South Audley Street
London W1Y 5DQ
Tel: 071 499 7532

IRELAND
The Ulster Cancer Foundation
40-42 Eglantine Avenue
Belfast BT9 6DX
Tel: 0232 663281/2/3
Helpline 0232 663439 (9.30-12.30 weekdays)

Irish Cancer Society
5 Northumberland Road
Dublin 4
Tel: 0001 681855
or dial 10 and ask for 'Freephone Cancer'
(Ireland only)

USA
American Cancer Society
Tower Place
3340 Peachtree Road, NE
Atlanta
GA 30026

Cancer Information Service
Building 31
Room 10A24
9000 Rockville Pike
Bethesda
MD 20892
Tel: 800 4-CANCER

National Cancer Survivors Network
PO Box 4543
Albuquerque
NM 82196
Tel: 505 268 7388

Papanicolaou Cancer Center
PO Box 016960
Miami
Fl 33136
Tel: 800 4-CANCER

USC Cancer Center
1721 Griffin Avenue
Room 205
Los Angeles
CA 90031
Tel: 800 422 6237

AUSTRALIA
Australian Cancer Society Inc
GPO Box 4708
Sydney
NSW 2000
Tel: 02 211 2599

Cancer Information and Support Society
65 Bay Road
Waverton 2060
Tel: 922 2334

Index

INDEX

205